Transcultural Midwifery Practice

Concepts, Care and Challenges

Transcultural Midwifery Practice

Concepts, Care and Challenges

Edited by

SARAH ESEGBONA-ADEIGBE, BSc (Hons), MSc, PGDip Health Research, PGCHE, RN, RM, FHEA
Senior Midwifery Lecturer/Course Director
Institute of Health and Social Care
Midwifery Division
London South Bank University
London, UK

ELSEVIER

Notices

Practitioners and researchers must always rely on their own experience and knowledge in evaluating and using any information, methods, compounds or experiments described herein. Because of rapid advances in the medical sciences, in particular, independent verification of diagnoses and drug dosages should be made. To the fullest extent of the law, no responsibility is assumed by Elsevier, authors, editors or contributors for any injury and/or damage to persons or property as a matter of products liability, negligence or otherwise, or from any use or operation of any methods, products, instructions, or ideas contained in the material herein.

ISBN: 978-0-3238-7230-0
Printed in India
Last digit is the print number: 9 8 7 6 5 4 3 2 1

Content Strategist: Poppy Garraway
Content Project Manager: Arindam Banerjee
Design: Brian Salisbury
Marketing Manager: Austin OSaben

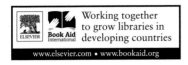

Working together to grow libraries in developing countries

www.elsevier.com • www.bookaid.org

CONTENTS

Transcultural Concepts in Midwifery

INTRODUCTION

In this chapter, you will explore the underlying theories and models which can be utilised for effective transcultural midwifery care. An overview of the key concepts of culture, cultural competency and cultural safety will be provided in relation to midwifery practice. The impact of immigration and acculturation and how this may impact on individual women will be included. This chapter ends with a discussion on the importance of cultural competency and cultural safety for midwives and the impact of this on optimum pregnancy outcomes for women from diverse backgrounds.

The Theory of Culture

WHAT IS CULTURE?

Culture means different things to different people and on a day-to-day basis we think that we know what culture is. However, when you delve into the intricacies of culture, it is a very complex phenomenon. Throughout the years, there has been many theories developed around what defines culture and various textbooks will provide different definitions and different theories of culture. Despite these various definitions, more or less the same aspects are stated that culture is a different way of doing things by different groups of people. The term culture is derived from the Latin word 'colere', which means to tend to earth and grow.

DEFINITION OF CULTURE

Helman (2007) defines culture as a set of guidelines that individuals inherit as members of a particular group, which influences how the world is viewed emotionally and their behaviour in relation to other people and the natural environment. The inheritance factor within Helman's definition suggests that culture is learned behaviour; however, where we learn this behaviour from will differ from individual to individual. A multidisciplinary consensus definition provided by Singer et al. (2016, p. 242) is that culture is 'an internalised and shared schema or framework that is used by group (or subgroup) members as a refracted lens to "see" reality, and in which both the individual and the collective experience the world'. This definition pinpoints the subjective and objective view of culture. To clarify, an individual may view their culture differently to other individuals from the same culture. The lens through which the individual views their culture is unique.

Eliot (2010) discusses three senses of culture: culture of the individual, which relies on the culture of the group, and the culture of the group which relies on the culture of the society. The influence of society on the group and the influence of the group on the individual are deciding factors on how culture is transferred. It can be confusing for midwives when faced with several definitions of culture. A simpler way to look at culture is to suggest that it is a way that people live their lives within the community in which they live and within the society in which they live.

It is stated that culture encompasses age or generation; gender; sexual orientation, occupation and socioeconomic status; ethnic origin or migrant experience; and religious or spiritual beliefs (Nursing Council of New Zealand, 2011; Hollins, 2018). Individuals do not need to be located in a particular place for a culture to be maintained as tradition passes down from generation to generation customs, beliefs and practices of long standing (Esegbona-Adeigbe, 2011). Therefore, culture is sustained provided there is an individual to continue these practices. Women who have migrated to other countries would therefore most likely continue to practise and maintain their culture.

THREE LEVELS OF CULTURE

Culture has three levels, a tertiary level that is visible to the outsider, the secondary level of culture which includes the underlying rules and guidelines not generally relayed to outsiders, and a primary level which is hidden (Hall, 1984). The tertiary level of culture may provide clues to midwives of the culture of a woman due to the language she speaks and her mode of dress. The secondary level of culture is not as visible as the tertiary level but may be realised by midwives who have regular or continued contact with women from that culture. Certain behaviour or practices may be evident to midwives as coming from a particular culture such as the woman performing cultural rituals.

The primary level of culture includes rules that are known and obeyed by all and may be almost unconsciously performed; it is more stable and the most resistant to change (Hall, 1984). The primary level of culture may not be visible even to midwives who have regular or continued contact with women from that culture, due to the hidden nature of rules and behaviour which are not often verbalised but inherent. The primary level of culture presents a challenge in the provision of health services as unawareness of this level may create unseen barriers. However, some midwives may have insight into primary levels of culture if they have in-depth knowledge of the culture leading to increased cultural awareness and sensitivity.

An analogy of a plant can help explain the levels of culture

The Primary Level of Culture

The seed of the plant is the primary level of culture. It contains the information that forms a culture. The nature of a seed is that information is hidden and it is difficult to determine what nature of plant will develop from it. This seed contains all the cultural practices and traditions that have been passed down from generation to generation. This information is privy only to those who are born into the culture. This hidden culture is private and secret and rarely spoken about to outsiders. Examples of this are inherent respect for elders, family and community and culturally acceptable methods of communication.

The Secondary Level of Culture

The roots that materialise from the seed may begin to illustrate to an outsider the nature of the plant, however, identifying the plant is difficult until tendrils begin to emerge above ground level. This may be compared to culture whereby some parts are exposed to outsiders due to the fact that they are visible. For instance, individuals from some cultures perform common rituals that are continued although they have become westernised or are living in foreign societies. These rituals may be the observance of cultural festivals and celebrations.

The Tertiary Level of Culture

The plant that will eventually be established from the seed is visible to all and is easily identified which is like the tertiary level of culture. Individuals from cultures may be identified if they maintain their traditional dress, eat their traditional foods and listen to their traditional music. An outsider can identify with this variation and see what makes this culture different from others. Hence, the culture may be distinguishable and more easily classed.

Exercise

Think about a woman who is booking for antenatal care. What levels of culture do you think may be visible during the booking interview? What information about her culture would you need to ask her to determine her views on care in pregnancy?

Practice Point

Reading the description of the levels of culture highlights some of the difficulties midwives may face when caring for a diverse childbearing population. Think about your primary level of culture that may not be visible to others. How would this impact on your interactions with healthcare services? In the next section, a broad overview of different cultures around the world is provided.

CULTURES ACROSS THE WORLD

Western Culture

Western culture includes the culture of European countries as well as those that have been heavily influenced by European immigration, such as the US (Zimmerman, 2017). Western culture has largely been influenced by Christianity in its early development. Today, the influences of Western culture can be seen in almost every country in the world (Zimmerman, 2017). Europe is a culturally diverse subcontinent. Individuals in different European societies differ in, among other things, their fertility patterns, lifestyles and rates of participation in preventive programs, and some of these variations may well be due to variations in attitudes, norms or other elements of culture. A large influence on European culture has been the migration of individuals from Africa and Asia impacting on food, dress and religion; this has been felt mainly in the UK. Migration has also impacted on North American culture; however, the historical impact of the transatlantic slave trade is also relevant.

Eastern Culture

Eastern culture generally refers to countries in Far East Asia (including China, Japan, Vietnam, North Korea and South Korea) and the Indian subcontinent (Zimmerman, 2017). Like the West, Eastern culture was heavily influenced by religion during its early development. In Eastern culture, there is less of a distinction between secular society and religious philosophy than there is in the West. Eastern religions lay the foundation for social and educational developments and shape the culture of the people. The common religions practised in the Eastern world are Hinduism, Buddhism, Jainism, Shenism, Taoism and Islam. The populations of Eastern countries are more traditional than people in the West, particularly in their clothing, rituals and so on. For instance, rituals such as Indians paying respect to their elders or parents by touching their feet and East Asians bowing as a gesture of welcoming guests, apologising and expressing thank you are common traditional practices.

Middle Eastern Culture

The countries of the Middle East have some things in common. The area consists of approximately 18 countries, including Bahrain, Cyprus, Egypt, Iran, Iraq, Israel, Jordan, Kuwait, Lebanon, Oman, Palestine, Qatar, Saudi Arabia, the Syrian Arab Republic, Turkey, the United Arab Emirates and Yemen. Most Middle Eastern countries are part of the Arab world. Arabs are the largest ethnic group in the Middle East, followed by Iranian peoples and Turkic-speaking people. The Arabic language is one thing that is common throughout the region; however, the wide variety of dialect can sometimes make communication difficult. Other popular languages include Persian, Kurdish, Hebrew and Turkish. Religion is another cultural area that the countries of the Middle East have in common. The Middle East is the birthplace of Judaism, Christianity and Islam. Most of the restrictions around pregnancy in Arab or Muslim women are related to religion. It is important to note that these are two distinct populations, one identified by religion and the other by ethnicity.

Caribbean Culture

Caribbean culture has been mainly influenced by European colonisation and the trans-Atlantic slave trade. The Caribbean is multicultural and very diverse. Officially, a quarter of the Caribbean population is English-speaking with Spanish being the next main language. However, there are 59 living languages spoken in the Caribbean (Paul, 2009). The Caribbean consists of 28 countries stretching from southeastern North America to northeastern South America. Cuba is the largest country in the Caribbean, followed by the Dominican Republic, Haiti, the Bahamas and Jamaica. The ethnic composition is very diverse in the Caribbean, consisting of people of indigenous, African and European descent, with different cultural traditions, which reflect the different colonising cultures. Many different religions are present in the Caribbean, including Christianity, Hinduism, Islam, Judaism, Rastafarianism, Buddhism and traditional African religions. This reflects the diversity of the population, which is also reflected in cultural practices which follow the ancestry of the individual populations.

African Culture

African culture has two influences, the indigenous tradition of Arab-Islamic and the European-Christian to which the continent has been exposed for well over a millennium. The values and lifestyles associated with these traditions have been assimilated and to a large extent indigenised on the continent (Arowolo, 2010). The continent of Africa is essential to all cultures. Africa is home to a number of tribes and ethnic and social groups. One of the key features of this culture is the large number of ethnic groups throughout the 54 countries on the continent. Nigeria alone has more than 300 tribes, for example. Currently, Africa is divided into two cultural groups: North Africa and sub-Saharan Africa. This is because Northwest Africa has strong ties to the Middle East, while sub-Saharan Africa shares historical, physical and social characteristics that are very different from North Africa. The harsh environment has been a large factor in the development of sub-Saharan Africa culture, as there are a number of languages, cuisines, art and musical styles that have sprung up among the far-flung populations. Africa is inhabited by various ethnic nationalities with their different languages, but despite their various cultures, Africans do share some dominant traits in their belief systems and have similar values that distinguish them from other peoples of the world.

Practice Point

A broad awareness of different cultures and their context is useful for midwives. Identifying where women are from and having some idea of the language they may speak and the religions they may practise is useful knowledge. However, care should be taken to explore with the woman her cultural background, religious affiliation and language, as assumptions can lead to miscommunication and misunderstandings. The next section discusses cultural diversity and how this varies within the individual and is dependent on several factors.

Cultural Diversity

Cultural diversity can be understood as the differences in colour, race, national origin, ethnicity, socioeconomic status, education, occupation, religion and other related characteristics of groups of people (Giger and Haddad, 2020). Cultural groups can share different characteristics but at the same time individuals are unique within these groups. Understanding that cultural diversity does not only relate to ethnic or cultural groups is an important point. Midwives may come in contact with women who have disabilities, who come from different socioeconomic backgrounds, who are lesbian, gay, bisexual or transgender and who have different educational status. Women may come from one ethnic background or have mixed heritage or have origins from several ethnic origins. Even if women are born into a particular culture, they may have been raised in another. Women may even practise a culture that is not related to their ethnicity.

Race refers to physical differences that women may identify with. Race is something that is inborn in our biology and is inherited across generations. Women may identify with one race or several, for example, African, Asian, European. A woman may consider herself to be black, brown or white, and it is important for the midwife to ask the woman what she identifies with. Ethnicity refers to common cultural characteristics such as language, practice and beliefs and is something that is acquired. No one is born with a language, for example, it is something that is learnt depending on the environment that they have lived in. The complexity of diverse cultures should not be underestimated, leading to the issue of how midwives tackle working with a diverse childbearing population. The next sections will discuss factors that impact on a woman's culture, but you should bear in mind that ethnicity, although a common factor in diversity, is not the only difference. 'Diversity' acknowledges 'differences in systems of shared' cultures and values. Although values, beliefs and practices could be shared in a 'culture', 'diversity' recognises the differences among single cultures and identifies characteristics that are autonomous and distinct (Dogra and Karnik, 2005). The challenges of midwives working with diverse cultures are never-ending but understanding what diversity can encompass is a great step in tackling this issue.

Acculturation

WHAT IS ACCULTURATION?

It is important at this point to look at acculturation, something that happens when groups from two cultures meet. Acculturation is typically the borrowing of traits from another culture, for instance, immigrants who arrive in a new country and adopt the behaviour of the dominant culture. It can also be argued that there may be influence of a less dominant culture on the dominant culture. A definition provided by Sam and Berry (2010) states that acculturation is the process of cultural and psychological change that occurs when two cultures meet. This may be a mixing of cultures or a dominance of one culture over another. Acculturation will occur differently for individuals, between groups and within society, and one cannot assume that acculturation occurs for every individual and if so to what extent.

It is significant to understand that acculturation does occur because the assumption could be made that cultures are sustained and do not change. However, with acculturation what may arise is a person adapting very quickly to the dominant culture or not changing their culture at all. In cases where there may be a mixing of the culture the extent to which this occurs may also vary within the individual. It is important to remember that the more contact an individual has with the dominant culture the greater may be the influence on their culture. However, if there is limited contact, then the acculturation may not occur to a high degree.

Acculturation Stress

The stress that results from cultural change is called acculturation stress. This stress can be positive if the individual enjoys being in a new country and looks forward to learning and adapting and may be negative if the individual is overwhelmed by all the changes (Kosic, 2004). Women, therefore, will adjust to being pregnant in a new country depending on the reasons why they have migrated. It is obvious that a woman who has been forced to migrate to a new country will have a different experience to a woman who has planned or wants to live a new life in another country. This can impact on her adjustment to a new healthcare service and her ability and desire to navigate maternity services. The factors that play a part in acculturative stress and the possible level of stress experienced by the individual are: similarities and dissimilarities between the two cultures, whether migration is voluntary or forced relocation and whether the contact is permanent (e.g., immigrant versus international student) (Beiser et al., 1993; Carballo, 1994; Berry et al., 1998; Kosic, 2004).

Acculturation stress can broadly be divided into two groups: features of the original and host society and individual characteristics and potential influence exercised by a number of demographic variables (Beiser et al., 1993; Carballo, 1994). Women are more likely to face different additional stresses during pregnancy depending on their marital status, education, country of origin and cultural, political and economic status. For instance, a woman who has family support, financial security and employment opportunities may be more likely to fare better in a new country than one who has little or no family support and financial security. If there are other issues which are political and economic in nature such as forced migration due to political or cultural issues then this can impact on the woman's experience.

The distance between two cultures, the country of origin and the host culture, is referred to as cultural distance. It has been found that the greater the difference, the more difficult it is for an individual to acculturate. Women who have migrated from one European country to another European or Western country may find the transition easier. This may not be the case for women who have migrated from Africa or Asia to a Western country where the cultures are likely to be widely different. Differences between cultures, among many examples, may include language and religion which can impact on the woman's ability to adjust to living in a new country and increase stress levels and impact on her mental health. The greater the cultural distance between two societies, the more likely that an individual will experience acculturative stress (Flores et al., 2011). When there are many cultural groups present in the host culture, the new society, it is known as a plural society. When the cultural groups are valued, it is known as a multicultural society. It is believed that migrants experience less stress in a multicultural society because they can maintain supportive cultural traditions (Flores et al., 2011). The UK has a multicultural society but how individuals are treated particularly in healthcare is an acknowledgment of valuing different cultures.

THE FOUR STAGES OF ACCULTURATION

There are two factors that influence acculturation, the extent to which individuals wish to maintain their heritage cultures and identities and the extent to which individuals wish to have contact with those from the dominant culture and participate with them in the daily life of the larger society (Sam and Berry, 2010). If there is contact with people outside of their culture, a person may not necessarily adapt their own culture and may still adhere to their usual cultural practices. Berry's (2006) (Fig. 1.1) model includes four types of acculturation strategies. The first type is integration. This is when the individual maintains his or her own cultural identity and at the same time participates in the host culture.

Individuals who integrate have an interest in maintaining their original culture but seek to be a member of the larger social network (Sam and Berry, 2010). You may come in contact with women who appear to have integrated well due to change in their dress, their employment/job role and their ability to navigate maternity services. These are all factors that demonstrate that the women may be adapting well to living in another country. Integration comprises acquiring identification with the host culture while maintaining identification with the home culture, also known

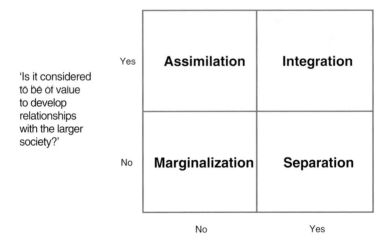

Fig. 1.1 Berry's acculturation model. (Adapted from Berry, 2006.)

as biculturalism (La Fromboise et al., 1993). There could be many factors that lead a woman to integrate but one reason may be that it is easier due to the need to engage in employment and education in the new country. Also important is if there are any language barriers as this will impact on integration due to the restrictions in communicating with the dominant culture.

Culture shock can occur with some individuals where there is personal disorientation when dealing with an unfamiliar way of life. Integration reduces the negative effects of culture shock and also lead to better psychological outcomes such as lower rates of depression (Virta et al., 2004). Women may feel less isolated if they integrate, especially if they are not living with family or close to communities who share the same culture as themselves. The adopting of both cultures leads to an ability to continue to practise their culture and provides the assurance that some cultural practices are maintained. Women may find this strategy more reassuring as they can acquire support from the new cultural groups but still seek support from their own cultural group.

Another type of acculturation is assimilation whereby the woman disregards her own cultural identity and becomes absorbed into the host culture. This is more likely to happen with younger individuals, often due to contact with other cultures through educational contact. In assimilation, individuals adopt the practices and outlook of the dominant culture and abstain from their culture of origin, often by seeking regular contact with the dominant society and avoiding maintenance of their original identity (Fox et al., 2013). This may lead to disconnection from family or friends. Women who assimilate may lose their support networks, however, it is possible that such support may be available in the host culture.

Berry (1994, 2010) discusses separation, the type of acculturation where the individual maintains his or her own cultural identity and rejects involvement with the host culture. Individuals who fall into the *separation* category are essentially the opposite of those who assimilate; they reject or avoid the new, dominant culture in favour of preserving their ethnic identity, often by highly valuing their original cultural practices and avoiding contact with dominant society individuals (Fox et al., 2013). Women who have language barriers or little social contact outside of their family and community are most likely to fall into this category. The reasons why women may separate could be voluntary or enforced. Voluntary separation could be due to fear of living in a new country and meeting different people, or be a personal value of adhering to cultural, spiritual or religious beliefs. Enforced separation could be due to issues such as domestic violence or slavery. The psychological health of individuals who adopt the separation strategy is said to be worse than individuals who integrate or assimilate (Berry, 1994). However, it is acknowledged that if separation is voluntary this can lead to less stress. You may possibly care for women who appear to be separated and it is necessary to explore why this has occurred to ensure appropriate support is provided.

Marginalisation is where individuals do not identify or partake in either their own culture or the host culture. The marginalisation strategy is defined as little possibility or lack of interest in cultural maintenance and little interest in having relations with others which could be due to reasons of exclusion or discrimination (Sheikh and Anderson, 2018). Marginalisation is often associated with negative outcomes, such as depression and lower self-esteem (Virta et al., 2004; Sawrikar and Hunt, 2005; Berry and Sabatier, 2010). Marginalisation may only apply to a small sample of migrants and studies have even suggested that this group is nonexistent (Unger et al., 2002; Schwartz and Zamboanga, 2008). This type of acculturation could also be as a result of failed attempts to assimilate probably caused by discrimination (Sam and Berry, 2006). It has been questioned by some that marginalisation is an impractical concept and that even in cases of discrimination, individuals are more likely to reframe their culture of origin rather than be left cultureless (Del Pilar and Udasco, 2004).

It was found by Sheikh and Anderson (2018) that higher educational status is associated with increases in identification with the host culture, independently of identification with the home culture. It is also suggested that individuals from a home culture with similar characteristics (e.g., language, quality of life, religion) to the host culture will be more likely to find the transition easier (Ward and Chang, 1997). Highly educated individuals are more likely to be integrated and, in some cases, assimilated (Sheikh and Anderson, 2018). The likelihood is that migrant women will attempt to settle in countries that have a cultural fit with their home country; however, often this choice may not be possible for some women. Integration has been considered the most adaptive mode of acculturation and has been associated with positive mental health outcomes (Lo, 2010).

Acculturation Strategies

Acculturation strategies depend on the extent to which the woman balances the two issues of culture maintenance and contact. It should be noted that the four strategies are not static and can change depending on situational factors (Sam and Berry, 2010). In addition, some women may adopt more than two cultures or be from two ethnicities making it difficult to adopt one acculturation strategy. A fixed focus on the acculturation of minorities implies that acculturation is something that happens only to minority people and that the cultures of dominant people are somehow unchangeable and without acculturative origins. This is not always the case, and you should realise that whether a woman belongs to a majority or minority culture both have an impact on each other. To suggest that minorities are psychologically reactive to intercultural contact and that dominant groups are not almost implies that minority people are a different species of psychological being, one distinct from the majority (Rudmin, 2003). Having an understanding of this point equips the midwife with some degree of awareness of the fluidity of culture and the opposite forces of the environment on individuals, organisations and societies in any cultural context.

Exercise

Review the two scenarios below to further understand the variations in acculturation.

Ayesha, a housewife, migrated to the UK 5 years ago. She lives with her extended family including her husband and three children. Ayesha speaks English and has adapted well to living in the UK; however, she only socialises in her community and does not have social contact outside of her family and close friends.

Farah, a healthcare worker in a care home, arrived in the UK 2 years ago and lives with her husband. Farah began working 6 months after she arrived in the UK and has developed a network of friends within her community and at work.

Learning Activity

1. After reading the two scenarios, state which stage of acculturation may have occurred for Ayesha and Farah?
2. What factors do you think may have influenced acculturation for Ayesha and Farah?
3. What factors would you need to consider if Ayesha or Farah were seeking pregnancy care?

Practice Point

Understanding that acculturation may occurs in different ways for migrant pregnant women you may care for is an important element in providing transcultural care. The midwife should understand how pregnant women may make health seeking decisions during pregnancy if they have migrated from another country. Another important element is acquiring cultural competency so that a midwife can understand a woman's cultural needs. This will be discussed in the next section.

Cultural Competency

WHAT IS CULTURAL COMPETENCY?

The term cultural competency was first devised by Cross (1989) as a 'set of congruent behaviours, attitudes and policies that come together in a system, agency or for professionals, to work effectively in cross-culture situations. Leininger (2002) first developed the concept of transcultural care in the 1950s and defined culturally competent care as the explicit use of culturally based care and knowledge that is used in sensitive, creative and meaningful ways to fit the general life ways and needs of individuals or groups for beneficial and meaningful health and well-being. The term cultural competency is commonly used interchangeably with cross-cultural or transcultural nursing (Fisher-Borne et al., 2015). As cultural competency consists of two sub concepts – 'culture' and 'competency' – definitions will vary depending on which part is the focus. If competency is the focus, the domains may be presented as knowledge or skill, whereas if the focus is culture then cultural values, religion and health beliefs are more specific (Shen, 2015).

The provision of culturally competent care is a multifaceted concept that incorporates not just factual knowledge of the customs, language and social norms of another culture, but some of reflection, self-awareness and cultural humility on the part of the healthcare provider (Tobin and Murphy-Lawless, 2014). Cultural competency is an important requirement in ensuring that midwifery care is effective. Papadopoulos (2006) states that the capacity to provide effective healthcare relies on considering people's cultural beliefs, behaviours and needs, which results in cultural competency. This view of cultural competency emphasises the importance of the woman's cultural perspective that should be integrated into healthcare provision.

Cultural competency, according to O'Hagan (2001), is an ability to maximise sensitivity and minimise insensitivity in health services. This is a simpler and more concise definition which does away with trying to identify any components that need to be incorporated into care to make such care culturally competent. Cultural competency in healthcare needs to include manifestations of the culture and competence components by domains or characteristics in affective, cognitive and practical/skill dimensions (Shen, 2015). The literature highlights that cultural competency consists of several theoretical components which are required; these will be reviewed in the next section.

THEORETICAL COMPONENTS OF CULTURAL COMPETENCY

Cultural Awareness

Cultural competency is said to begin with cultural awareness (Campinha-Bacote, 2008; Tomalin and Stempleski, 2013). A midwife who is not culturally aware is unable to work in a multicultural setting. Cultural awareness is the ability for a person to be aware that there will be differences between themselves and people from different backgrounds. If you are unable to recognise that there will be differences between your culture and the culture of the women, it can lead to negative behaviour and influences. Awareness of how culture, tradition and acculturation may affect individuals is the first step for midwives to understand a woman's cultural behaviour (Esegbona-Adeigbe, 2011). Awareness of these differences provides a platform for you to begin to discuss any differences in cultural rules or values. Cultural awareness requires self-examination and in-depth exploration of one's own cultural and professional background and involves the recognition of one's biases, prejudices and assumptions about individuals who are different (Campinha-Bacote 2008; Holland, 2018). A midwife who develops cultural awareness consciously approaches every contact with a woman differently.

Cultural awareness in midwifery practice should include knowing how women express themselves during pregnancy and how they deal with ill health. A midwife should be aware that although they will have undergone training on the normal physiology of pregnancy and how to detect deviations from the norm, women may have cultural expectations that impact on their views of pregnancy. Therefore, you should be conscious of perspectives outside of their worldview. Being culturally aware reduces the likelihood of making poor decisions and reduces compromising woman's care by making more considered decisions. It is vital for you to have cultural awareness not only for the woman but for your colleagues also. To begin to be culturally aware is to acknowledge what you do not know. It is also important to note that for you to be culturally aware does not mean compromising your own culture or sacrificing your own identity. The overall aim of cultural awareness is to increase respect for the woman and her family in all clinical interactions.

Cultural Knowledge

Cultural knowledge is the most important component of cultural competence for midwives to understand a woman's perspective (Esegbona-Adeigbe, 2018). Having knowledge of a woman's culture may allow a midwife to care more sensitively and appropriately for the woman. Healthcare professionals in the UK may have varying levels of cultural knowledge, and this may be dependent on their experience and level of education in this area. Midwives may gain cultural knowledge of specific groups of women if they work in an area where there is frequent contact. This cultural knowledge is learnt when caring for women and being exposed to their cultural practices. Holland and Hogg (2001) discussed the need to provide culturally appropriate and sensitive care and suggested the need for two levels of knowledge. The first level is for you to acquire expert knowledge in one or more cultures and the second level is for general awareness of various cultures. This knowledge can be acquired through training, education or experience with a culture in a variety of contexts (Foronda, 2008). Acquiring cultural knowledge may be opportunistic or something that is sought out by the midwife. Any cultural knowledge is expected to increase the midwife's ability to care for a woman. The difficulties arise when you are caring for a very diverse childbearing population in your clinical area making it difficult to acquire in-depth knowledge of any culture. However, in some cases some depth of cultural knowledge is possible in the context where a majority of women come from one particular background and you have frequent contact with this culture.

If a midwife achieves some depth of cultural knowledge, how this is utilised to care effectively for the woman requires additional skill from the midwife. Using cultural knowledge in clinical practice can lead to negative or positives outcomes. It is safe to say that each woman is unique, so any cultural knowledge needs to be used in a sensitive way. If cultural knowledge leads to stereotyping individuals this can lead to negative outcomes. No woman would wish to be provided care based on a midwife's experience with another woman of a similar culture. This means you need to know each woman on an individual basis and use cultural knowledge as a tool to initiate effective and useful discussions. If this is achieved, then you can build on existing knowledge of that culture but also take steps to ensure that the woman is receiving the care that she requires and needs. Cultural knowledge can also be used for improving communication with women whether they speak fluent English or not, as there are culturally acceptable ways of communication. In addition, cultural knowledge can provide you with the ability to adopt appropriate cultural behaviour depending on the context. It is always good to have cultural knowledge as a part of your skill set and every opportunity should be taken to build on this skill.

Cultural Encounters

Cultural encounters is the process that encourages midwives to directly engage in cross-cultural interactions with clients from culturally diverse backgrounds (Campinha-Bacote, 2002). This exposes the midwife to the norms and accepted behaviour of different cultural groups leading to increased knowledge of their culture. Cultural encounters is a pivotal component of cultural competency, as without this cultural awareness and knowledge cannot be developed. Some midwives during their practice who have encounters with various cultures on a daily basis will naturally acquire cultural awareness and knowledge. Other midwives who do not have these encounters or who regularly care for women from a similar cultural background as themselves may not develop their cultural awareness and in turn their cultural knowledge.

In an ideal world, part of midwives' training and practice should be compulsory cultural encounters. However, this is not realistic as the healthcare environment cannot be controlled to achieve this, but a cultural encounter can be achieved through experimental learning and simulation. Even if a midwife has the opportunity to care for women from diverse backgrounds, the quality of the encounter can be affected by the midwife's attitude. Open-mindedness is key as the cultural encounter is expected to modify the midwife's beliefs of the woman's culture and prevent stereotyping (Alizadeh and Chavan, 2020). In addition, open-mindedness allows the midwife to hear and consider new ideas and creates an ability to challenge personal values and beliefs. Lack of open-mindedness leads to the midwife not benefitting from the encounter.

Cultural Skill

A skill is the ability to do something well. So, it follows that cultural skill is the ability to engage with an individual from a different culture successfully. Cultural knowledge, awareness and encounters are required for a midwife to develop cultural skills. According to Campinha-Bacote (2008), cultural skill is the ability to collect relevant cultural data regarding the individual and how to conduct culturally based assessments. The focus here seems to be on adequate assessment of the woman; however, cultural skill is also the recognition that individuals may present their problems or concerns in a way that is different to yours and to assist this presentation, midwives should understand how this differs between women. It is also a crucial skill for understanding women's expectations when dealing with healthcare services. A midwife who has developed the cultural skill in assessing women is more likely to acquire vital information that may not have been divulged to other healthcare professionals. Such information could be vital in achieving an optimum pregnancy outcome. Therefore, the need for cultural skill should not be underestimated.

Cultural Desire

Cultural desire is said to underpin the entire process of cultural competence (Isaacs et al., 2016). A midwife without the desire to learn about other cultures will mostly have limited knowledge of different cultures despite having clinical interactions. Cultural desire is the motivation of the healthcare provider to want to, rather than have to, engage in the process of becoming culturally aware, culturally knowledgeable and culturally skilful and desire to have cultural encounters (Campinha-Bacote, 2002; Campinha-Bacote, 2008). Lack of cultural desire means midwives will not engage or seek opportunities to explore different cultures. In addition, lack of motivation may prevent you from accepting differences and being open to learning from women and exploring their culture. Campinha-Bacote (2002) suggests that without the desire to be culturally sensitive, cultural competence training might not be useful. A midwife cannot be forced to have cultural desire; hence, it is a skill deficit that cannot be overcome by any amount of training.

The building blocks of cultural desire are caring, love, sacrifice, social justice, humility, compassion and social encounters (Campinha-Bacote, 2008). These elements also reflect some prerequisites for being a midwife, so it is hoped and expected that a midwife would have some cultural desire. It is believed that cultural desire is a skill that is learnt over a lifetime (Briscoe, 2013). Some midwives will have different degrees of cultural desire depending on their experience. Unfortunately, there are barriers including issues around racism and stereotyping that can impact on the degree of cultural desire. Therefore, training on attitudes around stereotyping, racism and discrimination is said to be more effective in achieving cultural desire. As commitment for cultural desire can also be affected by racism and discrimination then it follows that there is an impact on a midwife providing care for women. Campinha-Bacote (2008) suggests that developing cultural desire is difficult and that this desire is caught and not taught. Even with training it is difficult to assess a midwife's cultural desire as it is an intangible concept, which makes it difficult to measure (Isaacs et al., 2016). It is easier to see outward acts of cultural desire such as midwives seeking cultural encounters or cultural knowledge. To measure a midwife's internal cultural desire is impractical and impossible.

Cultural desire includes a passion and commitment to the process of cultural competence (Campinha-Bacote, 2003). It may be difficult for the midwife to deal with women who engage in behaviours that conflict with the midwife's personal values and belief. It is further suggested by Campinha-Bacote (2008) that the construct of cultural desire is spiritual caring and love, making it more important to some midwives depending on their spirituality and a personal belief that you should do good onto others.

Cultural Sensitivity

The provision of culturally sensitive care is a professional standard for midwives (Nursing and Midwifery Council (NMC) 2019) . It is not an individual choice to become culturally sensitive. The term cultural competency in the area of maternity care is deemed to mean that a person is sensitive to the sociocultural context of women and children in the provision of holistic care (Callister, 2005). Cultural sensitivity is really about acceptance of others. It is all very well to have cultural knowledge and cultural awareness but if there is no sensitivity, this can negatively impact on the midwife–woman relationship. Cultural sensitivity leads to respectful encounters with women and provides a platform for women to express their culture. Respect for cultures and traditions remains a fundamental requirement for midwifery (WHO, 2009; NMC, 2019). Midwives who respect their own cultural values but are able to adapt to the values of other cultures are deemed to be culturally sensitive.

Sensitivity to a woman's needs, although an important component of reducing cultural barriers, does not effectively meet all the cultural needs and wants of the woman. However, cultural sensitivity is important for you to be able to practise effectively when caring for women from other cultures. Midwives who have experience being with and supporting women from different cultures may have greater sensitivity because exposure helps individuals to internalise awareness of how other people live. There is a suggestion that the process of developing cultural sensitivity should be determined by a desire within professionals to become culturally sensitive (Campinah-Bacote, 2003, 2008). In addition, cultural knowledge and awareness are also prerequisites for cultural sensitivity. To be aware of differences allows you to adopt a sensitive approach to engaging with women. In addition, cultural knowledge equips you with an understanding of beliefs and values that need to be respected in interactions with women and their families.

Foronda (2008) performed a concept analysis of the term cultural sensitivity and uncovered attributes of knowledge, consideration, understanding and respect. These were preceded by diversity, awareness and encounters. Showing respect for a woman's culture encompasses interpersonal skills, verbal and nonverbal communication and embracing other cultures, languages and traditions. If a midwife does not respect a woman, this may lead to mistrust and less likelihood of the woman adhering to advice provided about her pregnancy. If a woman feels that she's being listened to by you, she would be more likely to respond positively to any advice. Using cultural sensitivity to ask thoughtful, respectful questions about a woman's culture or wishes is more likely to increase her confidence in you. Steps to making a woman feel valued could be achieved by sharing your own personal cultural views and beliefs with women and asking her about her beliefs and values. Culturally sensitive healthcare occurs when client expectations are aligned with healthcare provider's knowledge, attitude and behaviour (Doorenbos et al., 2005).

Although the responsibility for developing cultural sensitivity should rest with individuals, a process of critical reflection should be facilitated by good leadership (Briscoe, 2013). Organisations should facilitate cultural sensitivity training for midwives and encourage critical thinking to facilitate this. Self-assessment about cultural sensitivity should be part of the lifelong learning approach required for midwives after qualification (Briscoe, 2013). Cultural sensitivity training results in increased open-mindedness and cultural awareness, as well as improves understanding of multiculturalism and the ability to communicate with women from other ethnic minority backgrounds (Majumdar et al., 2004).

Cultural Humility

Cultural humility is defined as a lifelong process on self-reflection and critique, to redressing power imbalances and developing mutually beneficial partnerships with communities on behalf of individuals (Tervalon and Murray-Garcia, 1998). This statement means that you never reach a point where you no longer need to learn about culture. Thus, it should be a requirement for midwives to be flexible about looking at themselves critically and desiring to continually learn. Cultural humility processes also involve your self-awareness of personal and cultural biases as well as awareness and sensitivity to significant cultural issues of others (Yeager and Bauer-Wu, 2013). So, elements of cultural competency are evident here. Within this, the midwife should have a desire to fix power imbalances (Tervalon and Murray- Garcia, 1998). Once this is at the forefront of your aim during clinical practice, the basis for cultural humility is laid. It should be recognised that even though a midwife has professional knowledge of pregnancy, which the woman may not have, the woman has understanding outside the scope of the midwife (Waters and Asbill, 2013). Therefore, understanding the woman's context of pregnancy is essential.

A better understanding of the term cultural humility is gained by viewing what it is not (Foronda, 2008). This provides more clarity to midwives in determining if they are achieving cultural humility. Powerful words are noted in relation to cultural humility specifically when the opposite of it occurs such as prejudice, unconscious bias, intolerance, discrimination, stereotyping, exclusion, stigma, inequity, marginalisation, misconceptions, labelling, mistrust, hostility, misunderstandings, judgmental, undermining and bullying (Chang et al., 2012; Berg, 2014). For example, unconscious biases can have significantly negative consequences at all levels within healthcare organisations and can lead to barriers to women's care which impact negatively and affect health outcomes (Robinson et al., 2020). In order to practise true cultural humility, you should be aware of and sensitive to the historic existence of legacies of violence and oppression against certain groups of women (Sufrin, 2019). If the midwife is to build trust, exploration with a woman of the reason why she may have mistrust of healthcare services should be illuminated and made visible. There are various reasons for this mistrust including the history of racism, discrimination and more recent lived experience of disrespect at the hands of healthcare providers (Sufrin, 2019). It is believed that the process of cultural humility must be undertaken by the midwife as a process with women, communities and colleagues. To acquire cultural humility means to accept that cultural influences can change over time and that this depends on location. You need to be cognisant of any behaviour that affects the ability to achieve cultural humility. In Chapter 3, an in-depth exploration of barriers in transcultural care will be discussed as these are significant in the process of cultural humility.

Masters et al. (2019) discusses the 5 Rs as an important coaching framework required for cultural humility (Table 1.1). It is proposed that to achieve cultural humility, five steps should be undertaken by the midwife.

Each component of the 5 Rs has an ask and an aim and you must ask yourself if you agree with the aim. If in agreement, the midwife can proceed with reflecting on the associated question. Disagreement with the aim indicates tension and provides opportunity for internal exploration, as well as personal and professional growth, if the midwife chooses to investigate why disagreement with the aim exists.

Application of the 5 Rs can be used by leaders of maternity services in three ways according to Robinson et al. (2020). The first opportunity occurs at the individual level with acknowledging that everyone has unconscious biases. The second occurs during socialisation of new employees to the organisation and the third opportunity occurs when leaders sustain and promote a culture of reflection, such as with the 5 Rs practice (Robinson et al., 2020).

TABLE 1.1 ■ **The 5 Rs of Cultural Humility**

Reflection	Aim: I will approach every encounter with humility and understanding that there is always something to learn from the woman.
	Ask: What did I learn from each person in that encounter?
Respect	Aim: I will treat every woman with the utmost respect and strive to preserve dignity and respect.
	Ask: Did I treat everyone involved in that encounter respectfully?
Regard	Aim: I will hold every woman in the highest regard while being aware of and not allowing unconscious biases to interfere in any interactions.
	Ask: Did unconscious biases drive this interaction?
Relevance	Aim: I will expect cultural humility to be relevant and apply this practice to every encounter.
	Ask: How was cultural humility relevant in this interaction?
Resiliency	Aim: I will embody the practice of cultural humility to enhance personal resilience and global compassion.
	Ask: How was my personal resiliency affected by this interaction?

Reproduced with permission from Masters et al., 2019.

Cultural humility can be distinguished from cultural competency as the first term attempts to avoid any type of prejudice or discrimination, whilst the second term attempts to even out health disparities. It can be argued that the use of both approaches results in better health outcomes for service users. The midwife who achieves cultural humility as well as cultural competency is attempting to provide a high standard of care in any context. Women may not appear to be from diverse backgrounds but may suffer disparities in healthcare. Their differences may not be due to ethnicity but other factors such as sexuality, disability, socioeconomic status or educational status, for example.

Exercise

Please review the following scenario to increase your understanding of cultural competency.

Alison has been a midwife for several years and has experience of caring for women from different cultural groups. Alison has some cultural knowledge of caring for women from India and Africa. Her interest in caring for women from different cultures has arisen from a personal desire and Alison has continued to take an interest in any new cultures she may encounter.

Learning Activity

After reading this scenario, please discuss the elements that Alison is demonstrating that are important in acquiring cultural competency. What further activities could Alison undertake to further increase her cultural competency?

Exercise

Please review the following scenario to increase your understanding of cultural humility.

Alison has been caring for a woman from a middle Eastern culture. This is the first time Alison has had contact with this culture and has limited knowledge of any cultural beliefs and values the woman may have. However, Alison is aware that these beliefs and values may impact on the woman's behaviour and wants to work with the woman to understand this. In addition, Alison wishes to ensure that she cares for the woman with respect and dignity.

Learning Activity

After reading this scenario, please discuss the elements that Alison is demonstrating that are important in acquiring cultural humility. What further activities could Alison undertake to further increase cultural humility?

Practice Point

After reviewing the key components of cultural competency, you can see that there are important connections between each one. Consequently, the interdependent nature of the components is highlighted. You will need to acquire most of these components to become culturally competent. The next section will look at how each of these components have been utilised in cultural competency models.

Cultural Competency Models

There are several cultural competency models that can be utilised in clinical midwifery practice. This section will explore four cultural competency models and how they can be employed to provide culturally competent care. Cultural competency models are critical in making midwives practice more efficiently and effectively (Albougami et al., 2016). They are useful for providing a framework from which midwives can apply interventions to improve their interactions with women. Cultural competency models can also be utilised with any population (Raman, 2015). Therefore, the decision to utilise a model depends on the practitioner or organisation providing the healthcare. Currently, no cultural competency model is recommended by the UK NMC for midwifery practice. The NMC standards of proficiency for midwives states the importance of midwives obtaining cultural competence (NMC, 2019). Therefore, cultural competency is recognised as a key skill for midwives.

Cultural competence models can be categorised into theoretical models and methodological models (Shen, 2015). Both types of models place emphasis on only one component of cultural competence, either 'culture' or 'competency', with its domains presented explicitly leaving the characteristics of the other component discrete (Shen, 2015). Theoretical models see as, cultural competency as being a process or continuum and are based on concepts from other fields such anthropology, sociology and psychology, geography and political science (Shen, 2015). Theoretical models derive their domains directly from the attributes or definition of cultural competence. The focus of competency is dominant in theoretical models highlighting the domains of awareness, knowledge, skills and sensitivity.

Methodological model approaches focus on the methods that a professional might use to become culturally competent. The focus of methodological models is on the cultural component of cultural competency such as religion, values, beliefs and practices. In the next sections, four models will be discussed, selected for their simplicity and appropriateness for midwifery practice and for clinical interaction: two theoretical models by Papadopoulos et al. (1998) and Campinha-Bacote (2002), and two methodological models, one by Purnell (2002) and the clarification, utilisation, linking, turning, reviewing (CULTURE) model from Esegbona-Adeigbe (2018).

PAPADOPOULOS CULTURAL COMPETENCY MODEL

A theoretical model for developing cultural competency created by Papadopoulos et al. (1998) to provide effective healthcare consists of three factors: cultural awareness, cultural knowledge and cultural sensitivity (Fig. 1.2). This model highlights the different components required to achieve cultural competency and requires some level of self-awareness.

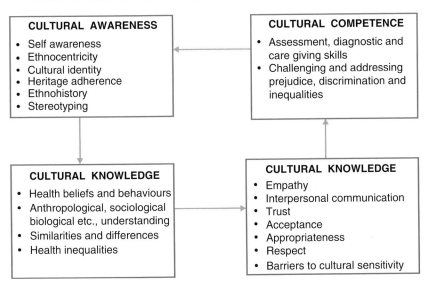

Fig. 1.2 Cultural competency model. (Reproduced with permission from Papadopoulos et al., 1998.)

A conceptual map is provided for each stage as a guideline. The first stage is cultural awareness which begins with an examination of personal values and beliefs, as it is important to have a cultural identity as well as realise influence on people's value bases and beliefs (Papadopoulos et al., 1998). The second stage is cultural knowledge of the anthropological (human behaviour), sociological (social behaviour) and biological nature of culture. Papadopoulos et al. (1998) states that the cultural sensitivity part of the model is achieved by involving women as equal partners. This leads to trust, acceptance and respect. The full state of cultural competence requires synthesis and application of previously gained awareness and sensitivity.

Papadopoulos (2006) also talked about developing culturally generic competencies which are applicable across different cultural groups or culturally specific competencies if caring for individuals from one culture. Cultural generic competencies include the appreciation of how cultural identity informs health seeking behaviour and how society and organisational structures promote or create barriers to culturally competent care. Cultural generic competencies are recognised by Papadopoulos (2006) as being useful for acquiring culturally specific care as shown in Fig. 1.3.

Depending on the circumstances in which the midwife is providing clinical care either a cultural generic or a culturally specific approach is required. For example, culturally specific knowledge would be appropriate for midwives who work with many women from a particular culture or ethnic group.

CAMPINHA-BACOTE MODEL OF CULTURAL COMPETENCY

The Campinha-Bacote model of cultural competency requires you to see yourself as becoming culturally competent rather than already being culturally competent and involves the integration of cultural awareness, cultural knowledge, cultural skill, cultural encounters and cultural desire, otherwise known as the ASKED model (Campinha-Bacote, 2002) (Fig. 1.4). This theoretical model reflects more than one contrasting world view (Higginbottom et al., 2011), and there is an interdependent relation between the elements. Campinha-Bacote (2002) states that the model begins and ends with cultural encounters and it is through these encounters that one acquires

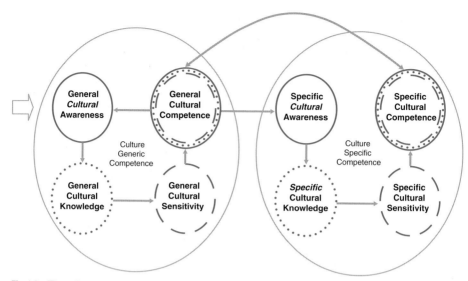

Fig. 1.3   The culture-generic and culture-specific model. (Reproduced with permission from Papadopoulos et al., 2003.)

cultural knowledge, cultural awareness, cultural desire, cultural skill and culture desire. Therefore, in this case, cultural competency is achieved by a continuous cycle of cultural encounters.

Campinha-Bacote (2018) further developed this model to consider cultural humility and changed the term cultural competency to cultural competemility. An intersectionality approach used in the model recognises the influence of organisational culture on individual culture (Campinha-Bacote, 2018). Cultural humility infuses each of the five constructs of cultural

Elsevier Ltd
125 London Wall
London
EC2Y 5AS
United Kingdom
t +44 20 7424 4200
elsevier.com

Registered office: The Boulevard, Langford Lane.
Kidlington, Oxford OX5 1GB, UK | Registered in
England, reg. no. 1982084 | vat no. 494 6272 12

14 October 2022

Dear Customer,

This notice is to make the reader aware that Elsevier has obscured figure 1.4 on page 18 of Esegbona-Adeigbe, Transcultural Midwifery Practice 1e, *9780323872300*. The figure was published without confirming the copyright holder's permission.

Please contact your regional Elsevier Customer Service representative with any questions.

Customer Service for Europe:
Europe, the Middle East and Africa: Tel: +44 (0)1865 844644 or to EurobkInfo@elsevier.com

Customer Service for other locations:
USA: Please contact Elsevier Customer Service with any questions at 1-800-545-2522 or www.elsevierhealth.com.
Asia-Pacific: Tel: +65 6349 0222 or to AsiaBKInfo@elsevier.com

We apologize for the confusion and/or inconvenience caused by this error.

Sincerely,

P Garraway

Poppy Garraway
Content Strategist

competency from an organisational and individual perspective (Campinha-Bacote, 2011). This model highlights the importance of cultural encounters, however, even with cultural encounters, the other components can be achieved by midwives through theoretical study and training.

PURNELL MODEL FOR CULTURAL COMPETENCE

The Purnell model is based on theories in biology, anthropology, sociology, economics, geography, political science, pharmacology and nutrition, as well as theories from communication, family development and social support (Purnell and Paulanka, 2003). This methodological model explores the different attributes of different cultures and sees cultural competency as a process not an end point (Purnell, 2002). This model is presented in the diagram (Fig. 1.5) with parallel circles that represent aspects of global society as well as community, family and person. There are 12 domains, which are heritage, communication, family roles and organisation, workforce issues, biological ecology, high-risk behaviours, nutrition, pregnancy, death rituals, spirituality, healthcare practices and healthcare professionals (Purnell, 2002).

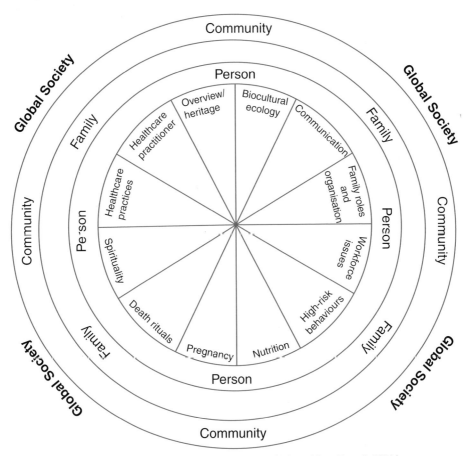

Fig. 1.5   Purnell model of cultural competency. (Adapted from Purnell, 2002.)

The Purnell model can provide useful insight into the aspects of the person's cultural needs in relation to each domain (Purnell, 2008).

1. Overview/heritage concerns country of origin, current residence and the economic, political environment. Consideration of reason for immigration is needed.

2. Communication relates to dominant language and dialects. It is also important to consider volume, tone and pace of voice, as well as non-verbal communication such as body language, facial expression and spatial distancing.

3. Family roles and organisation relates to gender roles, childbearing practices, role of elders and extended family members. Individual and family social status in community and views towards single parenting, childlessness and divorce are relevant.

4. Workforce issues relate to acculturation, assimilation, gender roles, communication styles and most importantly healthcare practices.

5. Biological ecology considers the racial and ethnic variation in physical attributes such as colour, body stature and the genetic, hereditary and endemic diseases manifestations as well as how drugs are metabolised.

6. Nutrition relates to meaning of food, food choices, rituals in eating, how food and food substances are used for health promotion, wellness and during illness.

7. Pregnancy and childbearing practices concern fertility, culturally accepted birth control, views of pregnancy and rituals and taboos that are said to harm or lead to a successful pregnancy.

8. Death rituals relate to how different cultures view death and behaviours that different cultures use to prepare for death and burials. Bereavement is also included.

9. Spirituality includes religious practices, use of prayer and behaviours that provide hope and comfort.

10. Healthcare practices include preventative and traditional, biomedical beliefs, as well as individual view towards mental health, chronicity, rehabilitation and organ donation. Response to pain and the sick are believed to be shared by culture. Barriers to healthcare are also included.

11. Health professionals' status and their perceptions of traditional beliefs and Western biomedical healthcare. The gender of the health professional is also important in some cultural groups.

The Purnell model recognises the global, societal and family influence on the individual. However, there are internal domains which influence the person's characteristics. Purnell developed his model initially for use as a framework for clinical assessment which is evident by the focus on nutrition, health behaviour, ill health and perceptions of ill health.

THE CULTURE MODEL

Esegbona-Adeigbe (2018), in a systematic literature review of cultural considerations in antenatal care, proposed the CULTURE model for cultural competency to reduce cultural insensitivity and maximise cultural awareness (Fig. 1.6). This model suggests that culture should be used as the first point of assessment for women when planning antenatal care (Esegbona-Adeigbe, 2011). The model recognises the key components of cultural competency from Campinha-Bacote (2002) and Papadopoulos et al. (1998) but is explicit at placing culture at the forefront of any midwife-woman/family interaction. Taking this stance allows you to acquire knowledge and utilise this to begin a plan of care for the woman. Although initially suggested for antenatal care, the CULTURE model can be used in the intrapartum and postnatal periods.

This model uses a methodological approach and begins with clarification of cultural needs, utilisation of this knowledge to initiate discussion on culture, linking information to health advice that may be required by the woman, turning advice into a care plan and reviewing care plan with

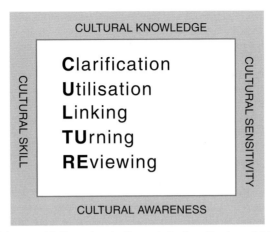

Fig. 1.6   Culture model. (Reproduced with permission from Esegbona-Adeigbe, 2018.)

women to ensure it is appropriate. This model provides the steps required to achieve cultural competency and requires the midwife to have some cultural awareness and pre-existing cultural knowledge to be able to initiate the conversation to explore the cultural needs of the woman. Cultural skill is required to utilise this information in considering the woman's care needs and develop a plan of care. Cultural sensitivity is required to enable the midwife to involve the woman in reviewing her plan of care.

A benefit of this model is the simplicity as well as providing an aide memoir for midwives. Often, important cultural information may be missed during midwife-woman interactions and if the woman is asked to review her plan of care this limits the incidence of missed information or miscommunication.

Practice Point

Cultural competency is multi-faceted and requires effective engagement by the midwife in order to acquire the necessary skills. Although cultural competency models provide a framework which midwives can utilise to provide more effective care the variety of models makes it difficult to decipher which is most appropriate.

COMPARING CULTURAL COMPETENCY MODELS

Each cultural competency model has positives and negatives in their appropriateness for midwifery practice. Shen (2015) and Capell et al. (2007) state that most models evaluate only the health professional's cultural competency with no consideration for the client and their health outcomes. Hence, the woman's views are not reviewed regarding the effectiveness of the cultural competency model utilised. The Papadopoulos et al. (1998) and Campinha-Bacote (2002) models have been validated, unlike the Purnell (Purnell and Paulanka, 2003) and the CULTURE (Esegbona-Adeigbe, 2018) models. This may guide a midwife to utilise one model over another. However, the practicalities of using a model will come down to personal preferences or organisational choice. The criticism of the Campinha-Bacote model is how health professionals can relate cultural knowledge to care provision and apply this to patient care. Midwives may face difficulty in trying to apply all elements of the Campinha-Bacote model to clinical encounters with women.

In addition, the domain of cultural desire may not be feasible for all midwives, mainly because as already discussed desire is very subjective and is multi-faceted. Desire could be authentic and genuine or missing due to other pressures making use of the model unachievable (Campinha-Bacote, 2003).

The main assumptions of the Purnell model of cultural competence involve looking at the broader perspective (Albougami et al., 2016). Critically, the Purnell and Paulanka (2003) model for cultural competence, and its associated framework involves drawing on a broader perspective, which makes it applicable to all healthcare environments and practice disciplines. However, the Campinha-Bacote model does hold more appeal because it helps to address cultural competency with respect to healthcare delivery. The same can be said for the CULTURE model (Esegbona-Adeigbe, 2018) with respect to provision of culturally competent care in the immediate face-to-face interaction between the midwife and the woman. The Papadopoulos et al. (1998) model does discuss culture-generic competencies and how this leads to culture-specific competencies which is crucial and necessary for midwives who work regularly with particular ethnic groups of women. This is a useful aspect for midwives as it provides a grounding of skills that can be further developed.

Brathwaite (2005) compared several transcultural nursing models using the following criteria: comprehensiveness, logical congruence, conceptual clarity, level of instruction, clinical utility and perspective. Only the Campinha-Bacote cultural competency model met all of Brathwaite's criteria. Theoretical and methodological models are both difficult to apply in any practice, therefore, more research is required to validate these models in midwifery practice.

Exercise

1. Think about how you can begin to increase your cultural competency in your clinical practice?
2. What component of cultural competency do you feel will be difficult to acquire?
3. How would you utilise any of the cultural competency models during midwifery practice?

Cultural Competency Training

Health policies, professional guidance and statutory requirements have encouraged cultural competency training (Workforce Race Equality Standard, 2015; NMC, 2019). However, on reviewing midwifery curricula and mandatory training in the UK it is not explicit that cultural competency training is addressed in a regular and persistent manner. In addition, evidence shows that cultural competency training is not configured so that midwives are adequately equipped with the knowledge and skills to translate this into midwifery practice. A review by George (2015) showed how the UK literature about 'cultural competence' is predominantly empirically, rather than theoretically, driven. Evidence suggests that current cultural competency training does not address the needs of culturally diverse groups, is delivered piecemeal and does not seem to be improving over time (George et al., 2015). As a consequence, the term cultural competency lacks conceptual clarity and rigour with regard to addressing cultural issues in practice when caring for a diverse population. This is worrying and impacts on whether healthcare organisations or higher education institutes prioritise cultural competency training.

Addressing health workforce cultural competence is a common approach to improving health outcomes for culturally and ethnically diverse groups (Jongen et al., 2018). It is already known that particular groups of women suffer adverse outcomes in pregnancy (Knight et al., 2019). Women from certain ethnic groups and lower socioeconomic status fare worse in pregnancy leading to the belief that their needs are not being met. Also, caring appropriately for women who are diverse in other ways, for example due to their sexuality and religion, is needed in midwifery practice. Therefore, cultural competency training should be incorporated into pre-registration midwifery training and mandatory training for qualified midwives. This should be included as an important element of training programmes and not just a tick box exercise. Cultural competence training has mainly concentrated on developing knowledge, awareness and sensitivity of individuals working in healthcare settings (Jongen et al., 2018). This is still good practice, but the literature reiterates the need to focus on teaching the skills needed to enable the practitioner to incorporate knowledge and awareness learnt into physical actions which can be applied and assessed in healthcare encounters and settings (Brach and Fraserirector, 2000; Hark and DeLissler, 2011; Dreachslin et al., 2012).

You can acquire cultural competency through clinical experience, but this will be dependent on the opportunities. As already discussed, midwives working mainly with women from similar backgrounds as themselves will unlikely be exposed to women and families with a diverse range of backgrounds. Hence, certain midwives may struggle with components such as cultural awareness or cultural knowledge. Cultural competency training evens the playing field for midwives regardless of what setting they work in. Some components of cultural competency training can be tailored to meet the requirements of midwives working with particular groups of women, such as cultural knowledge. Of course, care should be taken during any cultural competency training to stress the importance of not stereotyping women as this leads to inappropriate care for women who may not practise their culture in the same way. The approach of utilising cultural safety has been recommended as more likely to ensure women's cultural needs are being met. The next section explores the term cultural safety as it is important for you to see how cultural competency and humility are necessary in healthcare professionals, but the woman's cultural identity needs to be protected.

The Concept of Cultural Safety

WHAT IS CULTURAL SAFETY?

The concept of cultural safety has been around since the 1980s and was developed in New Zealand to cater for the needs of the indigenous Māori population (Ramsden, 1993). This was due to a need to reduce the health disparities experienced by the Māori people and improve their experiences when interacting with healthcare services. It was thought that this could be solved by addressing the cultural needs of the Māori people by changes in how healthcare was delivered.

Williams (1999, p. 213) states the concept of cultural safety as an 'environment that is spiritually, socially and emotionally safe, as well as physically safe for people; there is no assault challenge or denial of their identity, of who they are and what they need'.

The concept of cultural safety is relevant to pregnant women who should have a safe environment in which to give birth and have their preferences and needs met. Cultural safety involves protecting beliefs, practices and values of all cultures (Phiri et al., 2010). An important consideration for maternity service providers as when this protection is offered to women, this greatly improves their pregnancy and childbirth experience. It should be noted that the concept of cultural safety states that you should not focus on learning cultural customs of different ethnic groups but focus on being aware of difference, consider power relationships, implement reflective practice and allow the patient/woman to determine whether a clinical encounter is safe (Laverty et al., 2017; Curtis et al., 2019). In cultural safety, your self-awareness and the awareness of self-culture are more important than the awareness of the culture of the woman, because your own culture plays an important role in power inequalities in healthcare interactions (Curtis et al., 2019). It is natural that midwives assume power in the midwife–woman relationship due to the current provision of maternity care. Women leave their environment to enter the maternity service environment which is unfamiliar and is controlled by organisational policies and procedures. The inadvertent power over women that develops when they seek pregnancy care is a problem that can be diminished with cultural safety.

In order to further understand the concept of cultural safety, it is important that you revisit the concept of cultural competency. A key distinction between the concepts of cultural competency and cultural safety is the notion of 'power' (Curtis et al., 2019). Whereas the key distinction of cultural competency is cultural knowledge, cultural safety does not emphasise on the midwife developing cultural knowledge about the woman's culture even though this is an important component of cultural competency. The issue of describing and knowing the practices of other ethnic groups can lead to a checklist mentality that stereotypes group members (Desouza, 2008). This does not lead to meeting the woman's needs but rather may place her in a situation where she is being cared for inappropriately. In any case, the advantage of achieving cultural safety rather than cultural competency is that the former is a more realistic aim. Due to the wide diversity of the childbearing population it is impossible to acquire cultural knowledge for every woman you may care for. If the woman comes from a mixed ethnic background this further complicates the issue. In addition, a midwife having knowledge of a client's culture could be disempowering for a client who is excluded from their own culture (DeSouza, 2008).

The relevance of cultural safety is that focusing on your identity and increasing your awareness of this ensures that steps can be taken so that the woman's identity is not disregarded. Culturally safe healthcare professionals focus on self-understanding and the emphasis is on what attitudes and values they bring to their practice. A key principle is that a midwife who can understand his or her own culture and the theory of power relations can be 'culturally safe in any context' (Desouza, 2008). This is crucial in midwifery practice as midwives work with a variety of woman in a variety of settings. Having the ability to effectively care for women with different cultures, beliefs and values is a skill required to be an effective practitioner.

The midwife being able to recognise and protect a woman's cultural identity and therefore maintain their cultural safety is important, but organisational change is also relevant (Downing et al., 2011). Cultural safety is also concerned with both systemic and individual change with the purpose of enhancing health workers' awareness of their own identity and its impact on the care they provide to individuals from different cultural groups (Downing et al., 2011). The essence of cultural safety is emphasis on organisations recognising the social, historical, political and economic circumstances that create power differences and inequalities in healthcare and the clinical encounter with the woman (Kirmayer, 2012). Once this is in place, then women can experience maternity provision that is aligned to her health needs and personal preferences. A woman should have a voice in how she is cared for during pregnancy in any setting and once this is achieved then cultural safety is achieved.

THE NEED FOR CULTURAL SAFETY IN MATERNITY CARE

As previously discussed, the NMC standards of proficiency for midwives states the importance of midwives combining clinical knowledge, understanding and skills with interpersonal and cultural competence (NMC, 2019). This is not a unique recommendation, as in the past, national policies and guidance have also included an emphasis on cultural needs of women in maternity care. Historically, reports such as the National Health Service (NHS) plan and the National Service Framework (Department of Health (DOH, 2000; 2004)) highlighted that healthcare services needed to acknowledge a person's cultural beliefs in order to improve access. Maternity Matters, a report which focused on providing choice to women during pregnancy, stated that services should be accessible to all women and be designed to take a full account of their individual needs, including cultural needs (DOH, 2007). The Royal College of Gynaecologist and Obstetricians (RCOG) maternity care guidelines that focused on women with social needs also recognised cultural needs of women and encouraged cultural sensitivity to motivate vulnerable and hard-to-reach women to engage with maternity services (RCOG, 2008).

In the report Midwifery 2020, the importance of integrating cultural competency in midwifery training was stated as an important component of midwives' skills (DOH, 2010). National Institute of Clinical Excellence (NICE) guidance for women with complex social factors were developed, as women still did not understand the healthcare system and how it worked and reported lack of cultural sensitivity from providers (NICE, 2010). This, again highlighted that, cultural competency in maternity care has continued to be an important aspect of providing high-quality care. Despite these recommendations women have still felt that their cultural needs are not considered, highlighted by a National Maternity Review commissioned to improve choice and safer care for women, which demonstrated that women still reported dissatisfaction with maternity services (NHS England, 2016). The relevant factors in this review were that women from different backgrounds felt that healthcare professionals needed to understand and respect their cultural and personal circumstances in order to improve their childbirth experience (NHS England, 2016). All of the aforementioned guidance and reports suggest that maintaining cultural competency in maternity services is an ongoing issue. Unfortunately, there is a lack of rigorous research interventions and practice interventions which are currently documented, of specific maternity interventions which are aimed to address culturally competent maternity services (Coast et al., 2014; Garcia et al., 2015; Jones et al., 2017). However, the incorporation of cultural safety also should be recognised as an intervention. The need to focus on cultural safety will achieve cultural competency and reduce the issues that may arise between the woman's culture and the midwife's professional and organisational culture.

CULTURAL COMPETENCY VERSUS CULTURAL SAFETY

There have been various opinions that lack of cultural competency has impacted on midwives practice (Hogan et al., 2018; Fleming et al., 2019). In one study, midwives believed that healthcare inequality among immigrants could be the result of miscommunication which may arise due to a shortage of meeting time, language barriers and different systems of cultural beliefs (Akhavan, 2012). Studies of midwives' views have also stated that improving midwives' cultural competency would better equip them to respond to the needs of an ethnically diverse population (Aquino et al., 2015). The common theme from these studies is the difficulties midwives encountered in meeting the cultural needs of woman and requirement for cultural knowledge. In another study on the reported barriers to supporting women with perinatal mental health, midwives stated lack of knowledge on cultural issues; lack of skill, in particular, skills to respond to a disclosure of a mental health issue; and fears of causing women offence and distress (Higgins et al., 2018). Also, in the absence of time, knowledge and support some professionals felt they were unable to develop their own cultural knowledge and skills or help migrant pregnant women to develop the competencies they needed to negotiate maternity care (Phillimore, 2016). Utilising cultural knowledge by midwives is not realistic against the background of other conditions women may present with.

In exploring women's views, Higginbottom et al. (2019) found that women with negative views perceived health professionals as insensitive to their cultural and social needs leading to avoidance of continuously utilising maternity care, illuminating the importance of creating an environment for woman that removes insensitivity even if there is limited cultural knowledge of their needs. Woman have also reported that they felt constrained in their ability to articulate their health or maternity needs to healthcare providers and disempowered in respect of their involvement in decision-making (Higginbottom et al., 2019). This highlights the important concept of cultural safety in reducing the power imbalance between the midwife and woman. If women feel disempowered, they are more likely to avoid situations where this occurs impacting on their health seeking behaviour. Incorporation of cultural safety into care provision for pregnant woman and training for midwives is a more appropriate concept to facilitate women's needs than attempting to overcome any deficiencies of cultural knowledge and skill.

Practice Point

Cultural competency is a desired skill for midwives. However, the skills required to achieve cultural competency may not be achievable by all midwives, especially cultural knowledge which can only be fully achieved with experience and contact with women from a particular culture. Complexities arise when a childbearing population is diverse and there may be numerous cultures making it difficult to acquire deep knowledge of all cultures. Cultural safety refocuses self-awareness of your own culture and an understanding of how this may impact on the woman.

MATERNAL MORTALITY AND MORBIDITY, INFANT MORTALITY AND LACK OF CULTURAL SAFETY

It is necessary to review how lack of cultural safety can impact on optimum pregnancy outcomes. The benefit of pregnancy care is the reduction in maternal mortality and morbidity, as well as reducing adverse neonatal outcomes. However, if women do not utilise maternity services as recommended then poorer pregnancy outcomes are inevitable. There has been an increase in maternal deaths for women from ethnic minority groups, for decades highlighting a problem that requires investigation (Centre for Maternal and Child Health Enquiries (CMACE) 2011); Knight, 2019; Knight et al., 2016, 2020). Poor or no antenatal care has been noted as a significant risk factor for maternal deaths in the UK (Knight et al., 2016, 2020 2021). Cultural factors have also been suggested by maternal mortality reports as one reason why women do not engage with antenatal care, but no further clarification has been provided. Cultural safety for women in relation to the antenatal care they access can be used to increase their engagement and satisfaction with antenatal care, thus increasing maternal and fetal wellbeing.

The maternal deaths between 2012 and 2014 in the UK compared to the previous triennium were significantly higher among women from black and Asian ethnic minority backgrounds compared to white women, showing a 4.19 relative risk (Knight et al., 2016). A quarter of these women were born outside the UK, arrived a median of 4 years before they died and 65% were from Asia and Africa (Knight et al., 2014, 2016). Additionally, women who had migrated into the UK within the last 4 years were predominantly at higher risk; suggestions for these findings have been vague and have only stated that this may be due to cultural factors implied in ethnicity with no further explanation (Lewis 2006; CMACE, 2011; Knight et al., 2016). Recent migration has not been defined in any maternal mortality reports, however a period of less than 4 years in the UK has been linked to maternal deaths since 2006 (Lewis 2006; CMACE, 2011). The possible links to women not feeling that maternity services meet their individual needs should not be ignored.

Cultural safety is crucial in not just reducing maternal mortality but also maternal morbidity. The odds of severe maternal morbidity are up to 83% higher for some ethnic minority women throughout all stages of pregnancy compared with white European women (Nair et al., 2014). The fact that the women survive pregnancy should not be deemed a positive outcome. Maternal morbidity can be just as devastating as a maternal death. The United Kingdom Obstetric Surveillance System (UKOSS) conducted a case study of 1753 women between February 2005 and January 2013. Findings showed that inadequate utilisation of antenatal services doubled a woman's risk of maternal morbidity; other factors were lack of information, language barriers or cultural differences (Nair et al., 2014).

The cultural differences women may experience can be overcome by practising cultural safety. The midwife can mitigate cultural differences and avoid reduced utilisation of antenatal care even if there are language barriers. Mental health issues in pregnancy have increased significantly in the UK. Lack of awareness about mental ill health, cultural expectations, ongoing stigma, culturally insensitive and fragmented health services and interactions with culturally incompetent and dismissive health providers all impact on ethnic minority women's ability to receive adequate perinatal mental health support in the UK (Watson et al., 2019). Again, the significance of dealing with the complexities of maternal conditions and cultural issues is highlighted. The ability to utilise cultural safety by midwives can overcome barriers to appropriate healthcare services.

Infant mortality is also another consideration regarding culturally safe antenatal services. It is debated by Puthussery (2016) that ethnic minority grouping regardless of migrant status is a significant risk factor for unfavourable outcomes for migrant mothers in the UK. An inability to access antenatal care leads to increased infant mortality in ethnic minority women (Houses of Parliament, 2016; (DOH, 2010). Maternal death resulting in death of the fetus is known to affect the educational and economic status of surviving children (CMACE, 2011; United Nations Population Fund (UNFPA, 2010); (WHO, 2016). The widespread impact of lack of culturally safe maternity care should take into consideration the long-term consequences of infant mortality on the family, community and country. The Mothers and Babies Reducing Risk through Audit and Confidential Enquires (MBRRACE) perinatal mortality report demonstrated variation in stillbirth rates across the country, despite controlling for deprivation and other factors meaning that all women were not receiving the best possible care (Knight et al., 2016, 2020). It is suggested by Gray et al. (2009) that a complex mix of deprivation and behavioural and cultural factors leads to a higher risk of infant death among black and other ethnic minority groups. Substantial ethnic disparity in risk of unexplained infant death exists in England and Wales, and this is not attributable to preterm birth or area deprivation and may reflect cultural differences in infant care. Similar themes of cultural differences and impact on care utilisation arise in causes of infant mortality, again leading to the importance of cultural safety and its effectiveness.

STRATEGIES FOR MIDWIVES TO ACQUIRE CULTURAL SAFETY

Cultural safety is based on your analysis of your cultural self and the impact this has on encounters with women (Phiri et al., 2010; Curtis et al., 2019). In the first instance, you should be aware that unsafe cultural practice comprises any action which diminishes, demeans or disempowers the cultural identity and well-being of an individual or does not recognise the cultural identities of individuals (Esegbona-Adeigbe, 2011; Holland, 2018). Cultural safety acknowledges the barriers to clinical effectiveness which arise from the inherent power imbalance between healthcare professional and patient (Laverty et al., 2017). Therefore, in improving the woman's pregnancy experience, you should recognise that providing care is influenced by your beliefs. Hence, the focus of cultural safety moves to the culture of the clinician or the clinical environment rather than the culture of the woman (Curtis et al., 2019). This stance then leads you to look consciously at your beliefs and how it impacts on your interactions with women.

Another consideration that you should take heed of is that it is the woman who judges whether the professional relationship feels culturally safe. Usually in maternity services more emphasis is on outcomes of pregnancy rather than how the woman views her pregnancy experience. Women will view any care provision as being culturally safe if they do not feel disempowered or overlooked when making choices in their pregnancy care. Cultural safety foregrounds power differentials within society, the requirement for health professionals to reflect on interpersonal power differences and how the transfer of power within multiple contexts can facilitate appropriate care arguably for all patients (Curtis et al., 2019). This calls for you to understand the bicultural nature of the midwife–woman relationship, beginning with yourself, your own race, culture and imprinted stereotypes, and seeking to understand the social determinants of health. Culturally safe care is achieved when there is no inadvertent disempowering of the recipient, where women are involved in the decision making and become part of a team effort to maximise the effectiveness of their care (Laverty et al., 2017).

Development of critical conscious is an essential skill for you in the development of cultural safety. Health practitioners, healthcare organisations and health systems need to be engaged in working towards cultural safety by utilising critical consciousness. To do this, they must be prepared to critique the 'taken for granted' power structures and be prepared to challenge their own culture and cultural systems (Curtis et al., 2019). Midwives are more likely to adopt practices that place them in a role of educator, advisor and advocating. However, this may place them in a position of power simply for the fact that they have more knowledge and skills of pregnancy care. Women are more likely to feel overwhelmed with information and advice during pregnancy and may often feel that the midwife 'knows best' and to go against any advice that may impact negatively on their pregnancy. You should be conscious of any power struggles which may not always be obvious in clinical encounters with women. Adopting this stance will open up discussions with woman on how they feel about their care provision and if they are satisfied. For you to begin to develop this critical consciousness involves training and sharing of culturally focused information on a regular basis.

The guiding principle in cultural competency training (CCT) is usually on equality as opposed to achieving optimal care for all patients, however, what is needed is a responsive programme that places individualised care at the centre of CCT and is clinically as well as politically informed (George, 2015). Midwives should see cultural competence as a representation of good clinical practice but should still regard each woman in the context of her own culture as well as from the perspective of their cultural values and prejudices. Hence, cultural competence training should not be restricted to knowledge of facts about other cultures that can result in further objectification and stigmatisation, but rather focus on developing an understanding of diversity and recognition of the multiplicity of issues that contribute to our understanding of culture (Tobin and Murphy-Lawless 2014). This understanding can then be utilised by the midwife to develop steps towards cultural safety.

In Chapter 2, the importance of transcultural communication will be explored and the strategies used to improve communication in clinical practice. In Chapters 3 and 4, exploration of religious and cultural beliefs and values and their importance will be undertaken and acknowledgement of how these may impact on midwives' clinical practice. In addition, professional and organisational culture will also be reviewed and how this impacts on the midwife's individual culture. The issues of discrimination and unconscious bias are important considerations in healthcare, as well as white privilege. These all present challenges in providing services that are equitable to all women. Cultural safety provides a decolonised model of communication, power sharing and negotiation and recognition of white privilege. Chapter 5, will explore the barriers to healthcare caused by discrimination, stereotyping, white privilege and unconscious bias and how these barriers need to be overcome to ensure women's pregnancies are not compromised.

Learning Activity

1. In your usual practice think about a time when you were caring for a woman who had a different culture. How did you become aware of this?
2. What are the main components of cultural competency models?
3. Think about a clinical encounter you have had with a woman where there may have been a power imbalance.

1. Why is it important to be aware of culture when caring for women and their families?
2. Why is cultural knowledge an important component of cultural competency?
3. What is the importance of understanding acculturation?
4. Why is it important that the woman decides if the care provided is culturally safe?

References

Akhavan, S., 2012. Midwives' views on factors that contribute to health care inequalities among immigrants in Sweden: a qualitative study. Int. J. Equity Health 11 (1), 47.

Albougami, A.S., Pounds, K.G., Alotaibi, J.S., 2016. Comparison of four cultural competence models in transcultural nursing: a discussion paper. Int. Arch. Nurs. Health Care 2 (3), 1–5.

Alizadeh, S., Chavan, M., 2020. Perceived cultural distance in healthcare in immigrant intercultural medical encounters. Int. Migr. 58, 231–254.

Aquino, M.R.J.V., Edge, D., Smith, D.M., 2015. Pregnancy as an ideal time for intervention to address the complex needs of black and minority ethnic women: views of British midwives. Midwifery 31 (3), 373–379.

Arowolo, D., 2010. The effects of western civilisation and culture on Africa. Afro Asian J. Social Sci. 1.

Beiser, M., Johnson, P.J., Turner, R.J., 1993. Unemployment, underemployment and depressive affect among Southeast Asian refugees. Psychol. Med. 23 (3), 731–743.

Berg, K.K., 2014. Cultural factors in the treatment of battered women with privilege: domestic violence in the lives of white European-American, middle-class, heterosexual women. J. Women Soc. Work 29, 142–152.

Berry, J.W., 1994. Acculturation and psychological adaptation: an overview. In: Bouvy, A.M., van de Vijver, F.J.R., Boski, P., Schmitz, P.G. (Eds.), Journeys into Cross-Cultural Psychology. Swets & Zeitlinger Publishers, pp. 129–141.

Berry, J.W., 2006. Contexts of acculturation. In: Sam, D.L., Berry, J.W. (Eds.), The Cambridge Handbook of Acculturation Psychology. Cambridge University Press, pp. 27–42.

Berry, J.W., Balls Organista, P., Chun, K.M., Marin, G. (Eds.), 1998. Readings in Ethnic Psychology. Taylor & Francis/Routledge, Florence, KY.

Berry, J.W., Sabatier, C., 2010. Acculturation, discrimination, and adaptation among second generation immigrant youth in Montreal and Paris. Int. J. Intercult. Relat. 34 (3), 191–207.

Brach, C., Fraserirector, I., 2000. Can cultural competency reduce racial and ethnic health disparities? A review and conceptual model. Med. Care Res. Rev 57 (1_suppl), 181–217.

Brathwaite, A.E.C., 2005. Evaluation of a cultural competence course. J. Transcult. Nurs 16 (4), 361–363.

Briscoe, L., 2013. Becoming culturally sensitive: a painful process? Midwifery 29 (6), 559–565.

Callister, L.C., 2005. What has the literature taught us about culturally competent care of women and children? Am. J. Matern. Child Nurs 30 (6), 380–388.

Campinha-Bacote, J., 2002. The process of cultural competence in the delivery of healthcare services: a model of care. J. Transcult. Nurs. 13 (3), 181–184.

Campinha-Bacote, J., 2003. Cultural desire: the key to unlocking cultural competence. J. Nurs. Educ 42 (6), 239–240.

Campinha-Bacote, J., 2008. Cultural desire: 'Caught' or 'taught'? Contemp. Nurse 28 (1–2), 141–148.

Campinha-Bacote, J., 2011. Coming to know cultural competence: an evolutionary process. Int. J. Hum. Caring 15 (3), 42–48.

Campinha-Bacote, J., 2018. Cultural competemility: a paradigm shift in the cultural competence versus cultural humility debate—part 1. Online J. Issues Nurs. 24 (1).

Capell, J., Veenstra, G., Dean, E., 2007. Cultural competence in healthcare: critical analysis of the construct, its assessment and implications. J. Theory Constr. Test. 11, 30–37.

Carballo, M., 1994. Scientific consultation on the social and health impact of migration: priorities of research. International Organization for Migration.

Centre for Maternal and Child Health Enquiries (CMACE), 2011. Saving mothers' lives: reviewing maternal deaths to make motherhood safer: 2006–2008. BJOG 118 (11), 1402–1403.

Chang, E.S., Simon, M., Dong, X., 2012. Integrating cultural humility into health care professional education and training. Adv. Health Sci. Educ. Theory Pract. 17 (2), 269–278.

Coast, E., Jones, E., Portela, A., Lattof, S.R., 2014. Maternity care services and culture: a systematic global mapping of interventions. PLoS One 9 (9), e108130.

Cross, T.L., 1989. Towards a culturally competent system of care: a monograph on effective services for minority children who are severely emotionally disturbed. CASSP Technical Assistance Center, Washington, DC.

Curtis, E., Jones, R., Tipene-Leach, D., Walker, C., Loring, B., Paine, S.J., et al., 2019. Why cultural safety rather than cultural competency is required to achieve health equity: a literature review and recommended definition. Int. J. Equity Health 18 (1), 174.

Del Pilar, J.A., Udasco, J.O., 2004. Deculturation: its lack of validity. Cultur. Divers. Ethnic Minor. Psychol. 10 (2), 169.

Department of Health (DOH), 2000. The NHS Plan—A Plan for Investment, A Plan for Reform. HMSO, London.

Department of Health (DOH), 2004. National Service Framework for Children, Young People and Maternity Services.

Department of Health (DOH), 2007. Maternity Matters: Choice, Access and Continuity of Care in a Safe Service.

Department of Health (DOH), 2010. Midwifery 2020. Delivering Expectations.

DeSouza, R., 2008. Wellness for all: the possibilities of cultural safety and cultural competence in New Zealand. J. Res. Nurs. 13 (2), 125–135.

Dogra, N., Karnik, K., 2005. Diversity training for psychiatrists. Adv Psychiatr Treat 11, 159–167.

Doorenbos, A.Z., Schim, S.M., Benkert, R., Borse, N.N., 2005. Psychometric evaluation of the cultural competence assessment instrument among healthcare providers. Nurs. Res. 54 (5), 324–331.

Downing, R., Kowal, E., Paradies, Y., 2011. Indigenous cultural training for health workers in Australia. Int. J. Qual. Health Care. 23 (3), 247–257.

Dreachslin, J.L., Gilbert, M.J., Malone, B., 2012. Diversity and Cultural Competence in Health Care: A Systems Approach. John Wiley & Sons.

Eliot, T.S., 2010. Notes Towards the Definition of Culture. Faber & Faber.

Esegbona-Adeigbe, S., 2011. Acquiring cultural competency in caring for black African women. Br. J. Midwifery 19 (8), 489–496.

Esegbona-Adeigbe, S., 2018. Cultural qualities and antenatal care for black African women: a literature review. Br. J. Midwifery 26 (8), 532–539.

Fisher-Borne, M., Cain, J.M., Martin, S.L., 2015. From mastery to accountability: cultural humility as an alternative to cultural competence. Soc. Work. Educ. 34 (2), 165–181.

Fleming, T., Creedy, D.K., West, R., 2020. The influence of yarning circles: A cultural safety professional development program for midwives. Women Birth 33 (2), 175–185.

Flores, L.Y., Mendoza, M.M., Ojeda, L., He, Y., Meza, R.R., Medina, V., et al., 2011. A qualitative inquiry of Latino immigrants' work experiences in the Midwest. J. Couns. Psychol. 58 (4), 522.

Foronda, C.L., 2008. A concept analysis of cultural sensitivity. J. Transcult. Nurs. 19 (3), 207–212.

Fox, R.S., Merz, E.L., Solórzano, M.T., Roesch, S.C., 2013. Further examining Berry's model: The applicability of latent profile analysis to acculturation. Meas. Eval. Couns. Dev. 46 (4), 270–288.

Garcia, R., Ali, N., Papadopoulos, C., Randhawa, G., 2015. Specific antenatal interventions for Black, Asian and Minority Ethnic (BAME) pregnant women at high risk of poor birth outcomes in the United Kingdom: a scoping review. BMC Pregnancy Childbirth 15, 226. https://doi.org/10.1186/s12884-015-0657-2.

George, R.E., 2015. Exploration of cultural competency training in UK healthcare settings: a critical interpretive review of the literature. Divers. Equal. Health Care. 12 (3), 104–115.

Giger, J.N., Haddad, L., 2020. Transcultural Nursing-e-Book: Assessment and Intervention. Elsevier Health Sciences.

Gray, R., Headley, J., Oakley, L., Kurinczuk, J.J., Brocklehurst, P., Hollowell, J., 2009. Inequalities in Infant Mortality Project Briefing Paper 3, Towards an understanding of variations in infant mortality rates between different ethnic groups in England and Wales, National Perinatal Epidemiology Unit, University of Oxford Department of Public Health, University of Oxford Retrieved from https://www.npeu.ox.ac.uk/downloads/files/infant-mortality/Infant-Mortality-Briefing-Paper-3.pdf

Hall, E.T., 1984. The Dance of Life: The Other Dimension of Time. Garden City, New York, NY.

Hark, L., DeLisser, H. (Eds.), 2011. Achieving Cultural Competency: A Case-Based Approach to Training Health Professionals. John Wiley & Sons.

Helman, C.G., 2007. Culture, Health and Illness, fifth ed. Hodder Arnold, Oxford.

Higginbottom, G.M., Richter, M.S., Mogale, R.S., Ortiz, L., Young, S., Mollel, O., 2011. Identification of nursing assessment models/tools validated in clinical practice for use with diverse ethno-cultural groups: an integrative review of the literature. BMC Nurs. 10, 16. https://doi.org/10.1186/1472-6955-10-16.

Higginbottom, G.M.A., Evans, C., Morgan, M., Bharj, K.K., Eldridge, J., Hussain, B., 2019. Experience of and access to maternity care in the UK by immigrant women: a narrative synthesis systematic review. BMJ Open 9 (12), e029478.

Higgins, A., Downes, C., Monahan, M., Gill, A., Lamb, S.A., Carroll, M., 2018. Barriers to midwives and nurses addressing mental health issues with women during the perinatal period: the mind mothers study. J. Clin. Nurs. 27 (9–10), 1872–1883.

Hogan, R., Rossiter, C., Catling, C., 2018. Cultural empathy in midwifery students: assessment of an education program. Nurse Educ. Today 70, 103–108.

Holland, K., 2018. Cultural Awareness in Nursing and Health Care: An Introductory Text. Routledge.

Holland, K.C., Hogg, C., 2001. Cultural Awareness in Nursing and Social Care: An Introductory Text. Arnold, London.

Hollins, S., 2018. Religions, Culture and Healthcare: A Practical Handbook for use in Healthcare Environments. CRC Press.

Houses of Parliament, 2016. Infant mortality and stillbirth in the UK. Retrieved from researchbriefings.parliament.uk

Isaacs, A.N., Raymond, A., Jacob, E., Jones, J., McGrail, M., Drysdale, M., 2016. Cultural desire need not improve with cultural knowledge: a cross-sectional study of student nurses. Nurse Educ. Pract. 19, 91–96.

Jones, E., Lattof, S.R., Coast, E., 2017. Interventions to provide culturally-appropriate maternity care services: factors affecting implementation. BMC Pregnancy Childbirth 17 (1), 267.

Jongen, C., McCalman, J., Bainbridge, R., 2018. Health workforce cultural competency interventions: a systematic scoping review. BMC Health Serv Res. 18 (1), 232.

Kirmayer, L.J., 2012. Rethinking cultural competence. Transcult. Psychiatry 49 (2), 149–164.

Knight, M., 2019. The findings of the MBRRACE-UK confidential enquiry into maternal deaths and morbidity. Obstet. Gynaecol. Reprod. Med. 29 (1), 21–23.

Knight, M., Bunch, K., Tuffnell, D., Shakespeare, J., Kotnis, R., Kenyon, S., Kurinczuk, J.J., on behalf of MBRRACE-UK. 2020. Saving Lives, Improving Mothers' Care – Lessons Learned to Inform Maternity Care from the UK and Ireland Confidential Enquiries into Maternal Deaths and Morbidity 2016–18.

Knight, M., Kenyon, S., Brocklehurst, P., Neilson, J., Shakespeare, J., Kurinczuk, J.J. (Eds.), on behalf of MBRRACE-UK, 2014. Saving Lives, Improving Mothers' Care – Lessons learned to Inform Future Maternity Care from the UK and Ireland Confidential Enquiries into Maternal Deaths and Morbidity 2009–12. National Perinatal Epidemiology Unit, University of Oxford, Oxford.

Knight, M., Tuffnell, D., Kenyon, S., Shakespeare, J., Gray, R., Kurinczuk, J.J. (Eds.), on behalf of MBRRACE-UK, 2016. Saving Lives, Improving Mothers' Care – Surveillance of Maternal Deaths in the UK 2012–14 and Lessons Learned to Inform Maternity Care from the UK and Ireland Confidential Enquiries into Maternal Deaths and Morbidity 2012-14. National Perinatal Epidemiology Unit, University of Oxford, Oxford.

Knight, M., Tuffnell, D., Kenyon, S., Shakespeare, J., Gray, R., Kurinczuk, J.J. (Eds.), on behalf of MBRRACE-UK, 2021. Saving Lives, Improving Mothers' Care – Surveillance of Maternal Deaths in the UK 2012–14 and Lessons Learned to Inform Maternity Care from the UK and Ireland Confidential Enquiries into Maternal Deaths and Morbidity 2017-19. National Perinatal Epidemiology Unit, University of Oxford, Oxford.

Kosic, A., 2004. Acculturation strategies, coping process and acculturative stress. Scand. J. Psychol. 45, 269–278.

LaFromboise, T., Coleman, H.L., Gerton, J., 1993. Psychological impact of biculturalism: evidence and theory. Psychol. Bull. 114 (3), 395.

Laverty, M., McDermott, D.R., Calma, T., 2017. Embedding cultural safety in Australia's main health care standards. Med J Aust. 207 (1), 15–16.

Leininger, M., 2002. Part I. The theory of culture care and the ethnonursing research method. Transcultural Nursing: Concepts, Theories, Research, & Practice. pp. 71–98.

Lewis, G., 2006. Saving Mothers' Lives: Reviewing maternal deaths to make motherhood safer: 2006-2008.

Lo, Y., 2010. The impact of the acculturation process on Asian American youth's psychological well-being. J. Child Adolesc. Psychiatr. Nurs. 23 (2), 84–91.

Majumdar, B., Browne, G., Roberts, J., Carpio, B., 2004. Effects of cultural sensitivity training on health care provider attitudes and patient outcomes. J. Nurs. Scholarsh. 36 (2), 161–166.

Masters, C., Robinson, D., Faulkner, S., Patterson, E., McIlraith, T., Ansari, A., 2019. Addressing biases in patient care with the 5Rs of cultural humility, a clinician coaching tool. J. Gen. Intern. Med. 34 (4), 627–630.

Nair, M., Yoshida, S., Lambrecht, T., Boschi-Pinto, C., Bose, K., Mason, E., et al., 2014. Facilitators and barriers to quality of care in maternal, newborn and child health: a global situational analysis through meta review. BMJ Open 4 (5), e004749. https://doi.org/10.1136/bjmopen-2013-094749.

National Health Service (NHS) England, 2016. Better Births, Improving Outcomes of Maternity Services in England, A Five Year Forward Plan. NHS England.

National Institute of Clinical Excellence (NICE), 2010. Pregnancy and Complex Social Factors: a Model for Service Provision for Pregnant Women with Social Complex Factors. NICE.

UK Nursing and Midwifery Council (NMC), 2019. Standards of proficiencies for midwives. NMC. Available at: https://www.nmc.org.uk/standards/standards-for-midwives/standards-of-proficiency-for-midwives/.

Nursing Council of New Zealand, 2011. Guidelines for Cultural Safety, the Treaty of Waitangi and Maori Health in Nursing Education and Practice. Nursing Council of New Zealand 2011, Wellington, New Zealand.

O'Hagan, K., 2001. Cultural Competence in the Caring Professions. Jessica Kingsley Publishers, London.

Papadopoulos, I., 2003. The Papadopoulos, Tilki and Taylor model for the development of cultural competence in nursing. J. Health Soc. Environ. Issues 4 (1), 5–7.

Papadopoulos, I., 2006. Transcultural Health and Social Care; Development of Culturally Competent Practitioners. Churchill Livingston, Edinburgh.

Papadopoulos, I., Tilki, M., Taylor, G., 1998. Transcultural Care: a Guide for Health Care Professionals. Quay books, London.

Paul, L.M. (Ed.), 2009. Ethnologue: Languages of the World, sixteenth ed. Dallas, Texas.

Phillimore, J., 2016. Migrant maternity in an era of superdiversity: new migrants' access to, and experience of, antenatal care in the West Midlands, UK. Soc. Sci. Med. 148, 152–159.

Phiri, J., Dietsch, E., Bonner, A., 2010. Cultural safety and its importance for Australian midwifery practice. Collegian 17 (3), 105–111.

Purnell, L., 2002. The Purnell model for cultural competence. J. Transcult. Nurs. 13 (3), 193–196.

Purnell, L.D., Paulanka, B.J., 2003. Transcultural Health Care: A Culturally Competent Approach. FA Davis, Philadelphia.

Purnell, L.D., Paulanka, B.J., 2008. Transcultural Health Care: A Culturally Competent Approach. FA Davis, Philadelphia.

Puthussery, S., 2016. Perinetal outcomes among migrant mothers in the United Kingdom: is it a matter of biology, behavior, policy, social determinants or access to health care? Best Pract. Res. Clin. Obstet. Gynaecol. 32, 39–49.

Raman, J., 2015. Improved healthcare and wellness outcomes in ethnically/culturally diverse patients through enhanced cultural competency in nurse educators. Online J. Cult. Competence Nurs. Healthc. 5, 104–117.

Ramsden, I., 1993. Cultural safety in nursing education in Aotearoa. Nurs. Prax. N. Z 8 (3), 4–10.

Robinson, D., Masters, C., Ansari, A., 2021. The 5 Rs of cultural humility: a conceptual model for health care leaders. Am. J. Med. 134 (2), 161–163.

Royal College of Gynaecologist and Obstetricians (RCOG), 2008. Standards for Maternity Care—Maternity Audit Indicators. RCOG.

Rudmin, F.W., 2003. Critical history of the acculturation psychology of assimilation, separation, integration, and marginalization. Rev. Gen. Psychol. 7 (1), 3–37.

Sam, D., Berry, J., 2010. Acculturation: when individuals and groups of different cultural backgrounds meet. Perspect. Psychol. Sci. 5 (4), 472–481.

Sawrikar, P., Hunt, C.J., 2005. The relationship between mental health, cultural identity and cultural values in non-English speaking background (NESB) Australian adolescents. Behav. Change 22 (2), 97.

Schwartz, S.J., Zamboanga, B.L., 2008. Testing Berry's model of acculturation: a confirmatory latent class approach. Cultur. Divers. Ethnic Minor. Psychol. 14 (4), 275.

Sheikh, M., Anderson, J.R., 2018. Acculturation patterns and education of refugees and asylum seekers: a systematic literature review. Learn. Individ. Differ. 67, 22–32.

Shen, Z., 2015. Cultural competence models and cultural competence assessment instruments in nursing: a literature review. J. Transcult. Nurs. 26 (3), 308–321.

Singer, M.K., Dressler, W., George, S., Baquet, C.R., Bell, R.A., Burhansstipanov, L., et al., 2016. Culture: The missing link in health research. Soc Sci. Med. 170, 237–246.

Sufrin, J., 2019. 3 Things to know: cultural humility. https://hogg.utexas.edu/3-things-to-know-cultural-humility

Tervalon, M., Murray-Garcia, J., 1998. Cultural humility versus cultural competence: a critical distinction in defining physician training outcomes in multicultural education. J. Health Care Poor Underserved 9 (2), 17–25.

Tobin, C.L., Murphy-Lawless, J., 2014. Irish midwives' experiences of providing maternity care to non-Irish women seeking asylum. Int. J. Women's Health 6, 159.

Tomalin, B., Stempleski, S., 2013. Cultural Awareness-Resource Books for Teachers. Oxford University Press, Oxford.

Unger, J.B., Gallaher, P., Shakib, S., Ritt-Olson, A., Palmer, P.H., Johnson, C.A., 2002. The AHIMSA acculturation scale: a new measure of acculturation for adolescents in a multicultural society. J. Early Adolesc 22 (3), 225–251.

United Nations Population Fund (UNFPA), 2010. Reducing Maternal Mortality. Human Rights Centre, University of Essex.

Virta, E., Sam, D.L., Westin, C., 2004. Adolescents with Turkish background in Norway and Sweden: A comparative study of their psychological adaptation. Scand. J. Psychol. 45 (1), 15–25.

Ward, C., Chang, W.C., 1997. 'Cultural fit': a new perspective on personality and sojourner adjustment. Int. J. Intercult. Relat. 21 (4), 525–533.

Waters, A., Asbill, L., 2013. Reflections on cultural humility. CYF News Retrieved from American Psychological Association website. Available at: www.apa.org/pi/families/resources/newsletter/2013/08/cultural-humility.aspx.

Watson, H., Harrop, D., Walton, E., Young, A., Soltani, H., 2019. A systematic review of ethnic minority women's experiences of perinatal mental health conditions and services in Europe. PLoS One 14 (1), e0210587.

Williams, R., 1999. Cultural safety—what does it mean for our work practice? Aust. N. Z. J. Public Health 23 (2), 213–214.

World Health Organisation (WHO), 2009. Global standards for the initial education of professional nurses and midwives. www.who.int/hrh/nursing_midwifery/hrh_global_standards_education.pdf.

World Health Organisation (WHO), 2016. The WHO application of ICD-10 to deaths during the perinatal period: ICD-PM. http://www.who.int/reproductivehealth/publications/monitoring/icd-10-perinatal-deaths/en/. Accessed August 1, 2017.

Yeager, K.A., Bauer-Wu, S., 2013. Cultural humility: essential foundation for clinical researchers. Appl. Nurs. Res. 26 (4), 251–256.

Zimmerman, K.A., 2017. What is culture? Available at: https://www.livescience.com/21478-what-is-culture-definition-of-culture.html.

Transcultural Communication

INTRODUCTION

Communicating across cultures requires adopting a shared language but also considering the woman's context. Throughout this chapter you will be encouraged to examine the basis of effective communication and the importance of communication with a culturally diverse childbearing population. Effective use of interpretation services and the issues that may arise are discussed. Exploration of effective versus ineffective communication will assist you in viewing how this may impact your midwifery care.

Communication Concepts

WHAT IS COMMUNICATION?

The word communication is derived from Latin and means to share and send and receive messages through verbal or nonverbal means. The person sending the information is considered the sender, and the person receiving the information is considered the receiver. It is imperative that the receiver gives feedback to the sender to inform the sender that they received all of the information the sender was trying to relay (Tennant et al., 2020).

Effective communication is crucial in developing interpersonal relationships in clinical practice (Bhat and Kingsley, 2020), and there are many ways you need to communicate, each of which plays an important role in sharing information. Culture influences how a person expresses their feelings and verbal and nonverbal communication (Giger and Haddad, 2020). The way you communicate reflects yourself and your background, and not everyone communicates in the same way. Hence, miscommunication can occur, and conveying of information can be hindered by misunderstandings and preconceptions.

Communication is an essential element of being a healthcare professional (O'Hagan et al., 2014). Midwives need communication to provide effective care and build relationships with women and their families. Another important aspect of communication within the field of midwifery is it allows you to appropriately provide the seamless and multidisciplinary care required by women and their families (Price, 2013).

The process of communication provides a method in which people can connect and is a continuous task utilising written or oral language, gestures, facial expressions and other symbols (Giger and Haddad, 2020). You will work with women from different cultures and backgrounds, highlighting the need to understand cultural differences and communicate sensitively (Papadopoulos et al., 2016). You should be aware of the cultural and social norms in communication to facilitate delivery and receive information during clinical practice effectively. This awareness includes cross-cultural communication involving verbal and nonverbal methods (Purnell, 2018). It is essential to understand that verbal, non-verbal, written and visual methods of communication are all affected by cultural values and norms.

Effective communication between two people requires overlapping verbal and non-verbal cues, either culturally specific or general (Baugh et al., 2020). Cultural influences arising from nationality, migration status, race, ethnicity, language, religion, age, gender identity, sexual orientation, socioeconomic status and educational attainment make culturally derived communication signals inherently more complex (McHugh, 1992; Baugh et al., 2020). There can be many nuances between sender and receiver, increasing complexity and giving mixed messages. The art of communicating sensitively with different cultures is a crucial skill to reduce the risk of poor care, mistrust of services, inappropriate treatments and poorer health outcomes for women.

VERBAL COMMUNICATION

Verbal communication is the use of language to transfer information through speaking or sign language. This type of communication is a common occurrence for midwives when providing pregnancy care. In the everyday practice of the midwife, verbal communication is the first method used to provide and retrieve information from the mother starting at the booking interview through to antenatal, intrapartum and postnatal care. Verbal communication in the first instance would usually appear to be effective in everyday interactions with women and their families. However, there are advantages and disadvantages to verbal communication. Take a moment to review these in Table 2.1.

After reviewing the disadvantages and advantages of verbal communication, it can be seen that several issues may arise when communicating information to women and their families. Therefore, understanding the factors can affect verbal communication is a good starting point in becoming an effective communicator. Only when this is realised can stances be made by the midwife to overcome any issues. One of the critical disadvantages of verbal communication is a language barrier, but even if this is not the case, you may face barriers in communication due to unawareness

TABLE 2.1 ■ **Advantages and Disadvantages of Verbal Communication**

Advantages	Disadvantages
Able to convey information quickly	Use of jargon and unfamiliar terms can hinder woman's understanding
Able to receive feedback from woman to determine understanding	Emotion or difficulty of topic can hinder expression or appropriate use of words
Able to pick up nonverbal cues	There may be a difference in perceptions and viewpoint
Flexible	Hearing or speech difficulties may impact on woman's understanding
	Language differences
	Cultural differences

of the importance of delivering information in a culturally sensitive manner. Issues may arise even if the woman has a good command of English due to culturally inappropriate communication. It is not simply enough to communicate with women but to be aware of the cultural norms of communication.

PARALANGUAGE

Verbal communication is not simply the articulation of words; other nuances are present. The term paralanguage includes variations in speech, such as voice quality, volume, speed of speaking, pitch, nonfluencies (e.g., uh, um, ah), laughing, yawning, hesitation noises, gesture and facial expression, etc. (Wilson et al., 2005; Riera et al., 2015). If you think about how you converse in everyday interactions, paralanguage is a normal part of speech. Wankhede (2013) distinguishes between language and paralanguage by stating that language refers to what is said, whereas paralanguage refers to how it is said. You should note that paralanguage differs between cultures. The woman, as well as hearing the words that you speak, will also see the messages conveyed by paralanguage. The same words may convey the same meaning; however, the volume, rate and emphasis placed on those words can change the meaning of those words (Wankhede, 2013). Therefore, in some instances, a woman may derive a different meaning from the advice she is given by a midwife, depending on which words the midwife has emphasised and the speed and tone of the information provided. A very light and gentle voice may be more acceptable than a firmer tone to some women. In some cultures, a low voice volume represents good social manners and a sign of higher education, whereas speaking loudly is a cultural norm in other cultures. In many cultures, voices are only raised when someone is angry or needs to express excitement (Al-Qaderi et al., 2017). The volume used by health professionals when speaking to their patients has been highlighted as an essential aspect of communication; for example, a raised voice during a consultation could create a negative impression (Kee et al., 2018).

SILENCE

You should also be aware of the significance of silence during verbal communication. Speech and silence have often been mistakenly viewed as having two exclusive functions. Unlike speech, which requires one's knowledge of a given language, silence is a universal language that could convey meanings understandable to all women irrespective of their language (Said, 2018).

Silence is maintained to express language and avoid disrupting communication (Said, 2018). Three causes of silence highlighted by Berger (2004) were unexpected information/deviant behaviour, extreme emotions and lack of information or knowledge. Silence has different meanings for different cultures. It should be noted that since humans are likely to misinterpret speech, they are more likely to misinterpret silence because silence is culture-dependent (Nakane, 2006) and is affected by factors such as beliefs, gender and speaking style.

In certain cultures, silence is used to express politeness and respect (McLaren, 2016). In some Western cultures, silence during a conversation is perceived as something negative that needs to be eliminated as soon as possible. In Arabian cultures, silence is characterised as something that implies privacy, whilst other cultures utilise silence to convey agreement between different groups (Li et al., 2017).

A woman may use silence in either way during clinical interactions; an important note you should take is not to assume that silence means that a woman has accepted any information you have given to her. Indeed, it may be that she is silent so as not to be impolite. Western healthcare practitioners must take caution in cross-cultural contexts not to misinterpret acts of nodding silence as signs of mutual understanding as these expressions could instead be masking confusion or suppressing emotions (Shahid et al., 2009). In addition, silence could mean that a woman is overwhelmed by the information she has received or is still trying to process the information. You can use silence in your communication to allow a woman time to respond or ask the woman if more time is needed to ask questions, especially if she needs to make decisions about her care.

VOLUME

The volume at which individuals speak can vary in different cultures. Volume conveys meaning that varies across cultures; for example, British English speakers use volume to convey anger, but Indian English speakers use loudness to command attention. African people may appear to speak loudly compared to Chinese people who may be softly spoken. Raising your voice is seen as a sign of sincerity in some cultures. Hence, if a woman comes from a culture where speaking loudly is a cultural norm, she may not realise that in other cultures, this conveys anger in some Western cultures.

LAUGHTER

The significance of laughter is also different in various cultures; Kirch (1979) stated that laughter in some cultures is regarded as a sign of amusement, but in Africa, it is sometimes used to express surprise, wonder or embarrassment. Humour can help healthcare professionals deal with the demands of work, foster good working relationships with colleagues and improve morale (Parums-Aug, 2015). Using laughter when communicating with women is not unacceptable, but you should be aware that this may be inappropriate in certain situations. If you have already built a relationship with the woman, you may already have some idea of how the woman will respond to laughter or jokes. If, for example, the woman uses laughter whilst communicating with you, then reciprocating may be appropriate as this shows you are listening and agreeing with her. A study of patients' perspectives on the use of humour in healthcare found that patients expressed a wish for healthcare staff to initiate and reciprocate humour (McCreaddie and Payne, 2014). So, some women may have no issues with this.

Learning Activity

Think about how you use silence in your verbal communication. Why did you use silence, and did you realise when?

Think back to when you have used laughter in your clinical practice when communicating with women. What response did you receive? Is there any time when you think laughter is inappropriate?

Practice Point

Being aware that there are cultural norms of verbal communication is essential knowledge for midwives. This creates a basis for you to begin to explore with the woman what is acceptable in her culture. Suppose you are unfamiliar with the woman's cultural norms. In that case, you may inadvertently offend the woman or make her feel uncomfortable by unintentionally communicating a negative message through culturally biased nonverbal communication. Cultural differences in nonverbal communication can be barriers to healthcare if midwives are not sensitive when interacting with women from different cultures.

NON-VERBAL COMMUNICATION

Nonverbal communication uses body language, gestures and facial expressions to convey information to others and can be used both intentionally and unintentionally. Verbal communication is complete and effective only when accompanied by suitable nonverbal cues (Bhat and Kingsley, 2020). Nonverbal communication is estimated to account for 60% to 90% of communication (Mehrabian, 1972; Lorié et al., 2017). In addition, nonverbal communication plays a significant role in fostering trusting provider-patient relationships and is critical to high-quality care (Lorié et al., 2017).

The absence of nonverbal communication impacts effective communication. For example, a recording of someone speaking does not provide facial expressions, so the listener would find it difficult to determine the speaker's mood. Facial expressions are an essential element of nonverbal communication. Extensive research suggests that the expressions of six basic emotions (happiness, sadness, anger, fear, disgust and surprise) are universal (Keltner et al., 2003). The relevance of universal expressions across cultures is that you can convey messages to women regardless of language barriers. Demonstrating the emotion of happiness, for example, is commonly used in clinical interactions. However, Yue (2005) states that nonverbal behaviour differs in meaning in different cultures. So, although many expressions are believed to have universal understanding, care still should be taken.

Nonverbal communication is an important skill that you unconsciously use in your everyday practice; it could be a smile when you enter a room to care for a woman or a touch to express sympathy and understanding. There are also advantages and disadvantages of nonverbal communication, which you should be aware of when communicating with women (Table 2.2).

On reviewing the advantages and disadvantages, it is possible to see how some aspects of nonverbal communication are helpful in midwifery practice; however, there are several cultural difficulties. A smile is an expression used in everyday communication to convey that a person is

TABLE 2.2 ■ Advantages and Disadvantages of Non-verbal Communication

Advantages	Disadvantages
Complements verbal communication by adding to its meaning, e.g., a pat on the hand to say you are sorry	Can be vague or imprecise, gestures may be mistaken for other meanings
Can, in some cases, be a substitute to verbal communication by use of gestures, e.g., holding your hand up to your ear to say you have difficulty hearing	Gestures may distort information that you are trying to convey
Gestures such as pointing can be used to reinforce verbal communication, like showing directions	Visual difficulties may impact understanding
	Language or cultural difficulties

happy to see another person. It is a sign of welcome and acceptance and may be used regularly by midwives in their interactions with women. A smile could also be misused when providing bad news to women, or if the woman is discussing a serious topic, a smile may make her believe that her views are not being taken seriously.

It is suggested that members of the same national or ethnic group may be more able to identify facial expressions (Elfenbein and Ambady, 2002). This is important in healthcare provision as culturally accepted nonverbal communication may be received differently depending on the cultural background of the midwife and the woman. Therefore, care needs to be taken to avoid conveying inappropriate facial expressions to different cultures. Some expressions are more likely to be interpreted in the same way in many cultures, such as anger, fear and disgust. Expressions of anger, fear and disgust would be inappropriate in most interactions, creating barriers to effective communication with women. Even though you may be conveying the appropriate words, the accompanying of inappropriate expressions is easily recognised by any woman regardless of whether she speaks English or not.

Body language can also be misinterpreted. Intercultural similarities and fundamental differences in body language are partly related to the use of the body language in its cultural context and its interpretation among people of that specific culture. For instance, the head movement to say 'yes' and 'no' is not similar in all cultures. Therefore, care should be taken that your body language does not convey a different meaning from what you are saying; in turn it is important to not interpret the woman's body language and assuming you know what she is thinking. In all instances, confirmation should be sought from the woman.

EYE CONTACT

Eye contact is important in many cultures; again, there are cultural norms that you should be aware of and their importance in communication. While many Western cultures regard people as being suspicious or shifty if they avoid eye contact with a partner in face-to-face conversation, in many Eastern and African cultures, downcast eyes are regarded as a sign of respect, which can lead to misinterpretation in the West (Al-Qaderi et al., 2017). However, in some Eastern, African and Caribbean cultures, meeting another person's eye can be perceived as rude or aggressive (Bauer, 2015). In one study, Asians were more likely than Westerners to regard a person who makes eye contact as angry or unapproachable and suggested that gaze direction (direct vs. averted) influenced perceptions about another person's temperament (Akechi et al., 2013). These findings signify that eye contact is socially determined, and awareness of this cultural norm is beneficial when caring for women.

It would be easy to make assumptions about a woman's psychological status if she has poor eye contact leading to a concern about her mental well being. On the other hand, a woman may believe that a midwife is not honest if there is poor eye contact. Eye contact is essential in non-verbal communication and is generally associated with honesty and candour (Bauer, 2015). Nonverbal behaviour has been found to affect perceptions about the truthfulness of a message, and the truthfulness of a message affects how much eye contact a messenger gives (Levine et al., 2006). Maintaining good eye contact with women is a good approach during communication, but care should be taken that this is not obtrusive and is a skill that you will develop over time. In a study of junior medical staff interaction with patients, lack of eye contact led to communication errors (Kee et al., 2018). Therefore, your approach should gauge the woman's amount of eye contact and mirror this, and if a woman has poor eye contact, continue to have a sufficient amount of eye contact.

NODDING

Nodding in different cultures has different meanings. The use of a nod to indicate 'yes' is a widespread practice in many cultures. In the Middle East, South and East Asia and most of Europe, a nod generally means that the person has accepted what you have said. Notably, in India, a 'head bobble' indicates that the person agrees or hears what you are saying. Therefore, caution should be taken in cultures where a single nod of the head could indicate 'no'. This is present in Greece, Turkey and Bulgaria, usually accompanied by a rolling up of the eyes and a sound similar to a tut (Kubilius, 2019). The cultural variations in nodding can lead to miscommunication and delivery of care to a woman that is not wanted. A stance to avoid this is to procure verbal acceptance from the woman rather than relying on her body language.

TOUCH

Everyday nonverbal communication practised during an appointment, such as speaking to the woman at a close distance or greeting the woman with a handshake, can be behaviours that certain cultures may find inappropriate (Li et al., 2017). Hua (2013) states that handshaking, in many cultures, is regarded as a polite gesture when people greet each other. It differs only in how firm it is. For example, in some countries, such as America, a firm handshake is expected, whereas in other countries such as China, a gentle handshake is more appropriate (Al-Qaderi et al., 2017). Muslims do not allow touch between different genders; it is regarded as impolite if a man attempts to shake hands with a woman and Muslim women may not shake hands with men (Al-Qaderi et al., 2017). Touch can take different forms and can have various meanings (Hull, 2016). Some other examples include patting the back and hugging. Touch can convey multiple emotions such as affection, sympathy, or familiarity (Hull, 2016). It varies depending on the person's intimacy, gender, age, status and cultural background.

IMPACT OF CULTURE ON COMMUNICATION

Culture is maintained and preserved by communication (Wang et., 2011). Without communication, many traditional practices would be lost. Cultural norms can impact expectations for specific nonverbal expressions within healthcare. For, example during the intercultural communication between Eastern and Western cultures, there may be some misunderstandings because of a different understanding of nonverbal behaviour (Al-Qaderi et al., 2017). Levine and Ambady (2013) examined the influence of nonverbal behaviour on racial disparities in healthcare and suggested that through historical minority group treatment and clinician disengagement, patient distrust can arise. Levine and Ambady (2013) also state that negative stereotyping and culturally bound nonverbal expectations can obstruct nonverbal communication and engagement in cross-racial patient-clinician encounters. Hence, in a midwife-woman encounter, nonverbal communication could be a hidden barrier to effective engagement during pregnancy care. Some midwives have developed the skill of when to use nonverbal communication. Due to the professional nature of the midwife's role, certain boundaries have to be maintained (NMC, 2018). However, gestures and touch to convey meaning or offer comfort may be used by midwives. The issue is understanding the woman's perspective and ensuring that any such gestures or use of touch does not cause offence.

Exercise

Review the scenario below to understand the importance of culture on communication further.

Sue has arrived for an antenatal booking interview and is having her first baby. When she is answering questions from the midwife, she makes little eye contact and appears nervous. The midwife finds it difficult to keep eye contact with Sue when asking certain questions and wonders if there are any underlying problems that she needs to be aware of.

However, after the midwife discusses the booking interview with a colleague, she is made aware that in the woman's culture, lack of eye contact is a sign of respect for people in positions of authority.

Learning Activity

After reading this scenario, one realises that assumptions may have been made about Sue's behaviour which may have led the midwife to plan to deliver care that would have been inappropriate. Think about how the midwife would have responded if she had been aware that lack of eye contact was a cultural norm with some women.

Exercise

In this next scenario, you will see how the midwife addressed these issues with Sue.

At the next antenatal appointment with Sue, the midwife asks her how she felt at the last appointment. The midwife reassures Sue that she is happy to discuss any concerns with her and that she is aware that it may be difficult for Sue, but that in the UK, it is expected that midwives form a relationship with woman and be supportive. The midwife emphasises that Sue is the person who is in control of the pregnancy, and any choices she makes will be facilitated if possible.

WRITTEN AND VISUAL COMMUNICATION

Communication can also be in visual and written formats. Due to the need to cater for a diverse childbearing population, it is necessary to provide written information in several languages. The issue arises when it is impossible to cater for every language of every woman presenting for maternity care. Often maternity units will provide translated material for the common languages spoken in their childbearing population; however, the likelihood is that a woman may present for care, and there is not suitably translated material. Phillimore (2016) found that information available in maternity units was produced in a small number of community languages, with the range of languages on offer not expanded despite the radical change of demographics in recent years and the emergence of some communities. Literacy was also assumed, leading to women being given written material in their languages that they could not read (Phillimore, 2016).

Some women may have a good command of English but may not be able to read English. In some cases, the woman may be able to read but not in the dialect she speaks. For example, in some East African countries, women are not taught to read in their dialect but may read Arabic as this is the language the Koran is written in. This highlights that you should not assume that she can read in a specific language if a woman speaks a specific language. Discussing this with the woman avoids her being provided with written material that is unsuitable. Provision of quality and accessible translated information in plain language and pictograms that take into consideration health literacy, such as the ability to interpret health information, would enhance the usability of health information and services by migrant women (Merry et al., 2011). The advantages and disadvantages of written and visual communication are presented in Table 2.3.

One of the key disadvantages of written communication is that emphasis on certain information cannot be made. Research has shown that many health information leaflets are poorly written and that most would be too complex for 43% of the English population (Protheroe et al., 2015); hence, the issues with the translation of these leaflets into other languages when there is already an underlying problem of poorly written information. Understanding written communication relies on the woman's educational status and her ability to understand medical terms. Women may have difficulty identifying medically significant complications, communicating their concerns effectively and taking an active role in their healthcare (Jonkers et al., 2011; Ward et al., 2019). In some cultures, verbal information is received more readily than written formats. This should be recognised by midwives who should ensure that when presenting women with written information, a general discussion of the key points should be undertaken, and any important aspects

TABLE 2.3 ■ **Advantages and Disadvantages of Visual and Written Communication**

Advantages	Disadvantages
Written communication can be produced in large numbers	Tone or brevity of communication cannot be reinforced in written communication
Visual communication can be used for illiterate individuals	Difficult to obtain feedback
Visual information can be used to deliver complex messages	Can be more costly to produce material
Written or visual information can be more flexible than verbal information and can be delivered in several languages	Language or cultural difficulties

within the document should be emphasised. Feedback is also important as this allows the midwife to explore the woman's understanding of the written material.

Other written methods of communication will also be an issue for women who have language barriers, such as internet resources. Studies show a strong association between health literacy, internet access and use; socio-demographic characteristics, particularly age, education, income, perceived health and social isolation and prediction of internet access (Estacio et al., 2019). Therefore, signposting women to internet resources may not always be feasible, particularly if there are language barriers. The use of television to convey important information to women can be useful. Many maternity units provide important information to women using the television format; again, if there are language barriers, translated content can be used. However, this can only cater to some women, as it may be impossible to provide translations for unusual dialects.

Exercise

Review the following scenario to increase your awareness of how to utilise written information.

Suraya is attending for an antenatal appointment. The midwife asks her about her baby's movements and provides her with an information leaflet about observing fetal movements after checking that Suraya is able to read the information.

At the next appointment Suraya asks the midwife if she should be concerned if her baby's movements have changed. After further discussion, the midwife realises that in Suraya's culture it is usual to discuss important aspects of healthcare verbally and not in written format.

Learning Activity

Think about how this situation could have been handled differently if the midwife had been aware of this cultural norm. In your practice, how do you present information leaflets to women, particularly those who may have a language barrier?

In the next scenario, review how the midwife communicates with a woman when relaying information about breastfeeding.

Exercise

Hana is attending for an antenatal appointment. The midwife discusses the benefits of breastfeeding with her and advises her of internet resources that she can utilise for further information.

Learning Activity

On reviewing this scenario, can you think of any possible problems that the midwife should have considered? What key information should the midwife retrieve from Hana before recommending any internet resources?

Communicating Verbally with Women

LANGUAGE

A language is a system of communication that consists of a set of sounds and written symbols used by the people of a particular country or region for talking or writing. Interaction with a language means you interact with culture. Language is complex and conveys thoughts, feelings, desires and intentions to others (Bonvillain, 2019). Of course, language varies between countries, within countries and within individuals who share the same language. Even skilled interpreters can find it difficult to convey complex emotions and concepts, as language is a way of looking at words, leading to misunderstandings.

Language and acculturation might also be possible barriers to effective communication, as a person's use of language can be influenced by different cultures (De Maesschalck et al., 2011). The obvious difficulties of understanding a woman whose language is different are one factor for midwives; however, several challenges may arise working with women from different cultures. There may be different frames of reference, and women may display their emotions and behaviours differently. The disadvantages of verbal and nonverbal communication both include language difficulties as an issue. When a woman is a fluent bilingual English speaker, it is important to be aware that communication issues can occur even when using a common language. Miscommunications even occur between individuals who speak the same language; a word's meaning may differ depending on culture and language background (Li et al., 2017).

It is also vital to remember that bilingual women may not know some medical terms in English. In addition, in some languages, some words used in the English language are not available. For example, the words 'thank you'; in many languages, there is no direct equivalent for 'thank you' (Schuessler, 2018). The social implications of saying thank you also vary across cultures; a phrase such as thank you is used for momentous favours. In other languages, for example, in Southeast Asia and West Africa, to say thank you frequently may seem strange or even insulting (Floyd et al., 2018). Interestingly, as there are many languages around the world where there is no word for 'thank you'. Offence should not be taken if a woman fails to thank you after receiving any care; what is more common are other expressions of gratitude.

Exercise

Think about a time when you misunderstood someone who had the same language as you.
    Imagine how hard it would be to get a full meaning when someone also has a different cultural background than your own.

Practice Point

A midwife should not assume that if a woman speaks English, she can understand any medical terms used in discussions about her care. It is important to explore with the woman her language needs and ensure that she has a complete understanding of any discussions.

USE OF INTERPRETERS

Eliminating language barriers is critical in assuring culturally competent care for women (Brooks et al., 2019). The acknowledgement of any language issues should be treated as a prime concern by the midwife. A professional interpreter is a best practice recommendation where language differences exist between clinicians, patients and families (El-Amouri and O'Neill, 2011; Douglas et al., 2011). Family members may thwart information, withhold information and not explain complex terms leading to more harm to the woman; in fact, having a family member interpret for you may be just as harmful as having no interpreter. A woman may find it difficult even with an interpreter to understand what you are discussing if the interpreter does not speak the same dialect or share the same cultural background. Additionally, interpreters may interject their own beliefs or assumptions in their discussions with women, thus thwarting the advice being given by the midwife. Often it is difficult for a midwife to determine if this is happening.

Using an interpreter may also have emotional repercussions due to the content of the encounter. This may be the case if the information is distressing, such as during discussions on bereavement or providing a poor prognosis. The use of male interpreters may also exacerbate women's discomfort about discussing their issues openly with the opposite gender, especially sexual health. Women in some cultures are not encouraged to discuss sexual health issues with men, let alone a male interpreter not known to them (Dune et al., 2017; Phillimore, 2016). Sexual health is positioned as shameful among some women from refugee and migrant backgrounds who cannot talk about sexual health with their husbands, let alone midwives and interpreters (Dune et al., 2017; Mengesha et al., 2018). For women seeking care, who have concerns about privacy and confidentiality, this may contribute to a women's reluctance to access care (Richters and Khoei, 2008). Some women have stopped attending appointments because the interpreter was male, or they knew the interpreter and were concerned about confidentiality (Phillimore, 2016; Crowther and Lau, 2019). All of these factors highlight that simply procuring an interpreter does not solve language barriers.

Developing the skill of working with an interpreter is crucial for midwives. It is not just simply a case of speaking as you would if the woman could understand English. One major issue that can arise during a consultation using an interpreter is that the message you wished to convey to the woman has not been delivered. Some other disadvantages are lack of speed as three people are in the consultation and it is a three-way conversation. There may be a misinterpretation of the information you have provided by the interpreter, which can lead to compromising the woman's care. However, the main issue is that the midwife is not proficient in using an interpreter, which may be more of a problem if telephone interpretation is used

There were three types of interpreters in a qualitative study on the role of interpreters for patients with low English proficiency (LEP) in an intensive care unit (ICU); see Fig. 2.1.

1. Verbatim interpretation – interpreters use literal interpretation;
2. Health Literacy Guardian – interpreters integrate advocacy into their role;
3. Cultural Brokers – interpreters transmit information incorporating cultural nuances (Suarez et al., 2021).

Verbatim interpretation describes a strict linguistic interpretation of the clinician's words. Most of the interpreters described their role as verbatim interpreters. Interpreters are comfortable in this role and rejected any modification or expansion of this role (Suarez et al., 2021).

A health literacy guardian role is important for alerting the midwife when communication and understanding might be threatened or unachievable. The importance of this interpretation role is making sure women and the clinical team understand each other, including intervening beyond standard interpreting during discussions.

In some cases, the interpreter may act as a cultural broker, a bridge between diverse cultures, with diverse beliefs, medical systems, preferences and ideologies. Interpreters view this role as a

There are recommended strategies for working effectively with an interpreter (Box 2.1).

BOX 2.1 ■ Best Practices for Working with an Interpreter

- Introduce yourself to the interpreter – This is important to assess the person's proficiency in English and professional training.
- Acknowledge the interpreter as a professional in communication.
- Speak directly to the woman, not the interpreter – The interpreter is the communication tool not the woman.
- Speak more slowly – Speaking more loudly will not get the message across more effectively.
- Speak at an even pace in short segments – Provide time for the interpreter to interpret, long segments may mean that important information is missed.
- Insist that every thing you say to the woman is interpreted.
- Do not hold the interpreter responsible for what the woman says or does not say – The interpreter is the medium not the source of the information.
- Be aware that there may be some medical concepts that have no linguistic equivalent in other languages – In this case pictures or diagrams may be useful.
- Give the interpreter time to restructure the information so that it can be presented in a culturally appropriate manner to the woman.
- Asking questions about traumatic, sensitive or personal experience should be explained as being part of the normal care and that information will be kept confidential.
- Avoid complex sentence structure, changing ideas in the middle of sentences and asking multiple questions at one time.

Adapted from Refugee Health TA. https://refugeehealthta.org/.

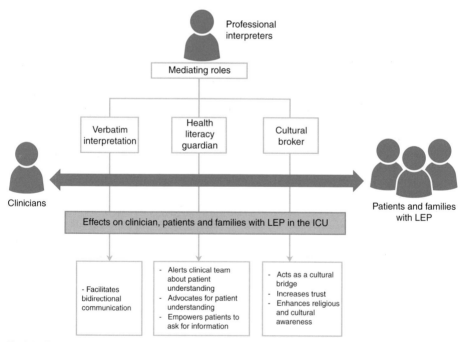

Fig. 2.1   Example of role of interpreters when working with patients with LEP in an ICU. ICU, intensive care unit; LEP, limited English proficiency.

way to 'breakthrough some of the cultural barriers' or to facilitate communication that incorporates background and women's habits and preferences (Suarez et al., 2021).

Types of interpreters: All three types of interpreters would be beneficial to midwifery practice; however, it could be argued that a health guardian literacy interpreter or cultural broker interpreter would facilitate more holistic communication with the woman.

Exercise

The next exercise reviews how the use of interpreters can be effective in midwifery practice.

Hana, who is attending for an antenatal appointment with her midwife, discusses the benefits of breastfeeding. The midwife is aware that as the interpreter is male and this may not be appropriate due to the issue of some cultures not discussing certain issues with individuals of a different gender. The midwife makes a decision to review this information at the next antenatal appointment and requests for a female interpreter.

Learning Activity

1. Discuss the issues here with the use of interpreters in communicating culturally sensitive information to women.
2. How else can a midwife overcome the possibility of barriers to culturally sensitive communication?

Cultural Display and Emotional Expression

CULTURAL DISPLAY RULES

Cultural display rules are cultural norms that govern the regulation of expressive behaviours depending on social contexts; these display rules can impact both nonverbal and verbal expressions (Matsumoto and Hwang, 2011). While taking cultural and linguistic differences into account, dealing with emotions is a complex challenge for health professionals (De Maesschalck et al., 2011). What is considered an appropriate display of emotion can differ from culture to culture. In some cultures, the display of anger, fear and frustration in certain situations is appropriate, whilst in other cultures, emotions are hidden. Subtle but definite differences in emotional expression are evident across cultures (Baugh et al., 2020). In Western cultures, high arousal emotions are valued and promoted; in Eastern cultures, low arousal emotions are valued (Lim, 2016).

In Table 2.4, you can see which emotions are attributed to high arousal and low arousal emotions (Russell and Pratt, 1980; Feldman, 1993; Tsai, 2007).

Culture determines how emotions are felt and expressed in a given context. It shapes the ways people should feel in certain situations and the ways people should express their emotions (Turner and Stets, 2005). Culture-specific display rules are learned during childhood, usually from parents. These culture-specific rules tell us whether it is appropriate to intensify, lessen, mask, or neutralise our emotional displays, as well as provide us with normative instructions for when and how to display our emotions (Pogosyan, 2015).

Cultural display rules are shaped by different cultural (e.g., the nation of origin), individual (e.g., family background) and environmental (e.g., societal gender norms) variables that shape people's behaviours, influencing emotion recognition and expression.

TABLE 2.4 ■ **High and Low Arousal Emotions**

High Arousal Emotions	Low Arousal Emotions
Anger	Bored
Excited	Depressed
Distressed	Calm
Happy	Miserable
Glad	Sleepy
Afraid	Dull
Fearful	Tired

TABLE 2.5 ■ **Six Main Classifications of Cultural Display Rules**

1. Having no effect, or emotion being expressed with no changes;
2. Exaggerating or expressing emotion with more intensity than internally felt;
3. Suppressing emotional expression than what is truly felt;
4. Masking or hiding emotions while expressing an emotion other than what they are feeling;
5. Neutralising emotional expression in situations where one might expect an expression; and
6. Qualifying emotions, by using verbal indicators such as, "No, I'm fine."

Reproduced with permission from Matsumoto, D., Yoo, S.H., Hirayama, S., Petrova, G., 2005. Validation of an individual-level measure of display rules: The Display Rule Assessment Inventory (DRAI). *Emotion* 5, 23–40. https://doi.org/10.1037/1528-3542.5.1.23.

Previous researchers have categorised cultural display rules into six main classifications in terms of how they affect emotional expression (Table 2.5) (Matsumoto et al., 2005).

Understanding that a woman's behaviour will vary between cultures and may be different from your own is essential for midwives. Some midwives may experience barriers in communication with a woman due to differences in cultural display practices. For example, expressiveness and verbalisation are valued highly in the Euro-American culture. Therefore, midwives from this culture may unconsciously expect this from women in their care. In contrast, some cultures, such as traditional Chinese and Korean cultures, tend to discourage the expression of physical and emotional distress to people outside of the family (Richters and Khoei, 2008). Hence, lack of expression or emotion may lead a midwife to assume an underlying issue in a woman who responds in this way, for example, when receiving bad news.

Exercise

Read the following example of how emotion may differ between women from different cultures.

Tina is attending for her 20-week scan and is informed that the baby may have a heart defect. She cries loudly and becomes very distressed. The sonographer calls a midwife to take her to a quiet room. On returning to the office the midwife discusses Tina's behaviour with her colleague and expresses her concern about her behaviour. Her colleague replies that it is not unusual for some woman from particular cultures to respond in this way to bad news.

Learning Activity

1. Take some time to think about how this situation could be handled in light of the information the colleague has supplied to the midwife.
2. What do you think are the difficulties for a midwife if women display their emotions?
3. What can be done to support other women in similar situations? Please review the following scenario for another example of cultural display.

Exercise

Sue is attending for her diagnostic test results and is informed that the results show that the baby has a congenital abnormality. The midwife is worried that Sue does not understand the results as she shows little emotion. She asks Sue if she understands the results, and Sue replies that she does. Her lack of emotion is unexpected, and the midwife is concerned that Sue may not have understood the diagnosis.

Learning Activity

1. On reviewing this scenario, think about the reasons why Sue is showing little emotion.
2. Are there expectations of women's behaviour when given the bad news that the midwife is unconsciously feeling?

After undertaking these two exercises, several points need to be considered. Hutchinson and Gerstein (2017) suggest that a critical aspect of clinical depression is the presence of depressed mood. Therefore, if you encounter a woman who has a low response or high response to information, you should explore whether this represents an actual depressive symptom, a norm learned in childhood, a coping mechanism, or a response to trauma. In addition, when working within a cross-cultural relationship, you should research cultural display rules and normative emotional expression specific to your client's culture.

Practice Point

After undertaking this exercise, it is important to consider that although cultural knowledge on emotional display would have been useful, the issue of cultural safety is more relevant here. Acknowledging that this is a cultural norm and not expecting the woman to adhere to the cultural expectations of the midwife or organisation is pivotal. You should not assume that behaviour is erratic or unusual, but take time to support the woman and ask questions about her feelings when it is appropriate. The display of no emotion can lead to the same assumptions as displaying intense emotion.

SPATIAL DIFFERENCES

The maintaining of proper distance when communicating with others is a cultural expectation. It is important to remember that we must maintain an appropriate distance when communicating with others—not too close, but not too far (Hull, 2016). Our personal space involves an invisible boundary surrounding our body. When our personal space is invaded, we react in a variety of ways as a manifestation of both our personality and our cultural background (Cai, 2019). The distance between two persons can be interpreted differently depending on various cultures (Bhat and Kingsley, 2020). For instance, it can either signify attraction or can signify intensity.

Maintaining a physical distance between people in conversation is also different from culture to culture (Mandal, 2014). Language of space can be classified as intimate space (within 45 cm), personal space (45 cm to 1.2 m), social space (1.2 to 3.6 m) and public space (3.7 to 4.5 m). People are very protective of their personal or intimate space. This personal space is generally reserved for our partners, family or close friends. When you speak to a woman, consideration of her personal space is paramount.

CULTURAL ETIQUETTE

Cultural etiquette includes codes of behaviour that rules different cultures. This, in other words, is simply having good manners which cross all cultures. Midwives who can demonstrate interest and respect for the women and families they care for are more likely to gain their respect and trust. In some cultures, asking about someone's health and family is required before getting down to the point. Individuals can take great offence if this is not done, but great appreciation may be achieved if this courtesy is given.

The simple point of saying hello and saying your name is another simple sign of being courteous. Some midwives pay great attention to social etiquette by asking the woman how she prefers to be called or taking great effort to pronounce her name correctly. In addition, introducing other professionals to women should also occur. Cultural awareness is a key skill in cultural etiquette.

CULTURAL TIMINGS

Western people structure their lives by milestones and deadlines; the inability to meet them could be interpreted as having a poor work ethic or being incompetent (Pant, 2016). This is known as clock culture, where the day is organised by the hours and minutes of the clock.

However, there are cultures that view time less importantly; emphasis is placed on doing things right and maintaining harmony, rather than worrying about getting things done 'on time' (Pant, 2016). In Western cultures, where there is reliance on the clock, the beginning and end of activities are strictly scheduled. However, in some cultures, scheduling is determined by the flow of activity or when the time feels right (Levine, 1997). Therefore, women's perception of time will be different depending on their culture. If a woman is late for an appointment, this may be perceived as disrespectful in Western culture, whereas in other cultures, if she is late, this does not raise concern. A woman who has recently migrated into a Western culture will need time to adapt to clock time.

Midwives Communication

COMMUNICATING SENSITIVELY

Clinicians are expected to have the knowledge and skills to communicate with service users in a culturally sensitive way (Betancourt et al., 2014). Midwives are assumed to have the requisite ability to communicate effectively with women during pregnancy. However, with the diverse childbearing population in the UK, many issues arise when achieving effective communication. Barriers can arise, impacting effective communication, including language issues, noise and distractions and biases; if this is overcome, cultural issues may appear (Fig. 2.2).

BARRIERS TO VERBAL COMMUNICATION

Culturally sensitive communication relies on midwives being able to critically reflect on their values, beliefs, preferences and culture and also have an understanding of traditions, perspectives and practices of culturally diverse individuals, families and communities (Douglas et al., 2011). A lack of culturally sensitive communication may mean that women and families are less likely to be

VERBAL COMMUNICATION

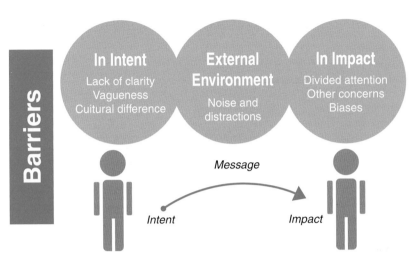

Fig. 2.2 Barriers to verbal communication. (Reproduced with permission from Counterproductive Communication: What Doesn't Work. A presentation at Heritage University at CBC Week 07, September 2019 in Pasco, WA 99301, USA by Jacob Campbell, https://presentations.jacobrcampbell.com/qXxd7D#sgb2bg3.)

satisfied with their care. There is an increased risk of miscommunication, and cultural disparities may result, leading to poor engagement with maternity services and poorer pregnancy outcomes (Betancourt et al., 2014; Paternotte et al., 2016). You can undertake key steps to achieving effective sensitive communication. However, communication does not solely comprise of giving information. It is vital that midwives recognise that active listening is a vital tool to be used in communication with women, families and colleagues (Price, 2013).

ACTIVE LISTENING

Active listening is the ability to listen to another person, respond and achieve mutual understanding. It is assumed that communication is just about talking, in which the midwife should be proficient since it is a key skill of clinical midwifery practice. However, the value of listening is a neglected concept in daily healthcare (van Dulmen, 2017). Midwives, on an everyday basis, educate, counsel and advice women about their pregnancy and care of their newborns. The ability to listen is just as important as talking and accounts for half of any conversation you may have with a woman. Listening is a communication technique that should require midwives as listeners to understand, interpret, count and evaluate what they hear from women.

An effective listener pays attention to cues like voice intonation, message length, emotion and body language (Tiwari, 2020). These elements provide additional information to the midwife when providing care to women and can be used to ensure a holistic assessment of her condition is achieved. Listening skills need to be developed by midwives; it does not just happen without effort. Many additional factors can get in the way of effective communication with a two-way communication process, and they can inhibit 'active listening'. You may face additional challenges when communicating with women from diverse backgrounds due to cultural differences.

The barriers affecting active listening by the midwife also impact the woman's becoming an active listener. Such barriers are especially prevalent among individuals with an inadequate or limited level of health literacy (Sorensen et al., 2015).

It is recommended that the following approach should be used for midwives to become good listeners (Tennant et al., 2020):

1. Focus on the sender
2. Listen to message and not you want to hear
3. Watch for sender's body language
4. Repeat back in your own words what you thought you heard the woman say
5. Clarify any questions
6. Do not make assumptions
7. Do not formulate a response until you have heard the whole message.

If you show the woman you are focusing on what she says, this reassures the woman that the information she provides is important. As well as observing the woman's body language, you should be aware of your body language. It is important to clarify what the woman has said to you and repeat what was said to the woman; this avoids common misconceptions. This is necessary even if an interpreter is being used. Avoiding assumptions is important as often this may lead to a woman being provided advice that is inappropriate or unnecessary.

ACHIEVING EFFECTIVE CULTURALLY SENSITIVE COMMUNICATION

Demonstrating Respect

Brooks et al. (2019) recommend demonstrating respect for the culture of the individual and their family by asking culturally sensitive questions about the patient's and family's values, beliefs and assessing the individual's psychological, physiological and sociocultural needs. In addition, questions about secondary languages and non-verbal communication techniques are also essential (Maier-Lorentz, 2008).

Developing a Trusting Relationship

Developing a trusting relationship with the woman and her family is essential. It can be achieved by using open and non-threatening body language to demonstrate a willingness to help and learn (Brooks et al., 2019). This creates a platform for the woman to open up during discussions. Establishing rapport and trust are critical elements to the communication process between you and the woman (Cross and Bloomer, 2010; Matteliano and Street, 2012).

ENCOURAGING THE WOMAN TO PARTICIPATE

It is important to involve and encourage women and families to participate in communication and decision making to the degree where they feel comfortable (Johnstone et al., 2016). The woman should be considered an important part of the team, and her views should be considered in all consultations.

Effective communication between maternity care providers and women in labour, using simple and culturally acceptable methods, is recommended by World Health Organization (WHO, 2018). Table 2.6 demonstrates steps that the midwife could use to ensure that communication with the woman and her family is culturally acceptable.

Using these methods not only demonstrates cultural sensitivity but facilitates cultural safety. These methods place women at the centre of care provision and protect their cultural identity.

TABLE 2.6 ■ Methods for Acceptable Communication

- Introducing themselves to the woman and her companion and addressing the woman by her name
- Offering the woman and her family the information they need in a clear and concise manner (in the language spoken by the woman and her family), avoiding medical jargon and using pictorial and graphic materials when needed to communicate processes or procedures
- Respecting and responding to the woman's needs, preferences and questions with a positive attitude
- Supporting the woman's emotional needs with empathy and compassion through encouragement, praise, reassurance and active listening
- Supporting the woman to understand that she has a choice and ensuring that her choices are supported
- Ensuring that procedures are explained to the woman, and that verbal and, when appropriate, written informed consent for pelvic examinations and other procedures are obtained from the woman
- Encouraging the woman to express her needs and preferences, and regularly updating her and her family about what is happening and asking if they have any questions
- Ensuring that privacy and confidentiality is maintained at all times
- Ensuring that the woman is aware of available mechanisms for addressing complaints
- Interacting with the woman's companion of choice to provide clear explanations on how the woman can be well supported during labour and childbirth

From WHO, 2018. WHO Recommendations on Intrapartum Care for a Positive Childbirth Experience. World Health Organization.

Exercise

The following exercise has been adapted from an effective communication strategy by Purnell (2018) and can assist midwives in understanding their communication practices.

Effective Communication Strategies for the Midwife (Purnell, 2018):

- Identify your cultural ancestry. If you have more than one cultural ancestry, choose one for the sake of this exercise.
- Explore the willingness of individuals in your culture to share thoughts, feelings and ideas. Can you identify any area of discussion that would be considered taboo?
- Explore the practice and meaning of touch in your culture. Include information regarding touch between family members, friends, members of the opposite sex and healthcare providers.
- Identify personal spatial and distancing strategies used when communicating with others in your culture. Discuss differences between friends and families versus strangers.
- Discuss your culture's use of eye contact. Include information regarding practices between family members, friends, strangers and persons of different age groups.
- Explore the meaning of gestures and facial expressions in your culture. Do specific gestures or facial expressions have special meanings? How are emotions displayed?
- Are there acceptable ways of standing and greeting people in your culture?
- Discuss the prevailing temporal relation of your culture. Is the culture's worldview past, present, or future oriented?
- Discuss the impact of your culture on your healthcare. Be specific, that is, not something that is very general.

Completing this exercise can increase your awareness of your communication style and related cultural norms. The usefulness of this activity can highlight to you any potential barriers to communicating effectively with women from other cultures.

Organisational Communication

In addition to the midwife's individual communication, the way an organisation communicates is also an important consideration in achieving culturally sensitive communication. Organisational structures, including hierarchy and significant power differences between midwives and other healthcare professionals, and healthcare policies influence the outcomes and satisfaction of women and families (Douglas et al., 2011). These power differences between health professionals can impact on the woman's care as poor communication policies can impact on the midwife's practice. If there is a hierarchy of power, the default may be that individuals in power have control over how policies are devised. What needs to be present is leadership that recognises the diversity of women attending pregnancy care and devise policies that guide midwives on acceptable practice.

Organisations need to ensure there are policies that are supportive of and enable culturally sensitive communication (Douglas et al., 2011). There is not only a need for policies that acknowledge cultural differences in communication but training and development of midwives to convey these practices into everyday clinical practice. An environment that cultivates effective communication practices needs organisational support through policy, resources and professional development opportunities to improve midwives' critical skills and knowledge related to culturally sensitive communication (Almutairi and Rondney, 2013). However, to ensure a healthcare service that is culturally sensitive and proficient, appropriate educational resources for midwives should also be available (Carroll et al., 2007).

Exercise

Review the following example from an organisation that took steps to improve culturally sensitive communication.

In East London, material that identified barriers to management of chronic health conditions was produced by the local hospital Trust to be used by the Bangladeshi population. This innovation process involved using interpreters to explore within the community reasons why they failed to engage with certain services and what barriers could be prevented. The result was that a culturally sensitive service through policy change and training was developed by the Trust in order to improve communication between health professionals and the Bangladeshi population.

Learning Activity

Think about how you can begin to increase culturally sensitive communication in your organisation.

What policies or training do you currently have in place in your organisations that could support midwives achieving culturally sensitive communication?

Are there any barriers in your organisation that affect culturally sensitive communication?

Practice Point

Culturally sensitive communication is the responsibility of maternity service providers and individual midwives. Recognising any barriers that impact the delivery of culturally sensitive communication is the first step. In addition, organisations need to support midwives in achieving good practice in culturally sensitive communication by creating policies and appropriate training. However, the individual midwife in everyday practice is ultimately responsible for delivering information to the woman and her family in a culturally sensitive manner.

REFLECTIVE QUESTIONS

1. What are cultural communication norms in your culture?
2. Do you think cultural norms in communication are different between midwives and women?
3. What do you think are the most useful steps a midwife can take to ensure effective communication with a woman?
4. Why do you think that there are barriers to culturally sensitive communication in maternity care?

References

Akechi, H., Senju, A., Uibo, H., Kikuchi, Y., Hasegawa, T., Hietanen, J.K., 2013. Attention to eye contact in the West and East: autonomic responses and evaluative ratings. PloS One. 8 (3), e59312.

Almutairi, A.F., Rondney, P., 2013. Critical cultural competence for culturally diverse workforces: toward equitable and peaceful health care. Adv. Nurs. Sci. 36 (3), 200–212.

Al-Qaderi, I., Alduais, A., Wang, S.L., 2017. Non-verbal communication across cultures: a case study of Chinese, Polish, Turkish and (Yemeni) Arabic cultures. Netw. Sci. J. Res. Result. Theor. Appl. Linguist. 3 (13), 53–62.

Bauer, R. 2015. The impact of making eye contact around the world. https://www.weforum.org/agenda/2015/02/the-impact-of-making-eye-contact-around-the-world/

Baugh, A.D., Vanderbilt, A.A., Baugh, R.F., 2020. Communication training is inadequate: the role of deception, non-verbal communication, and cultural proficiency. Med. Educ. Online. 25 (1), 1820228.

Berger, C.R., 2004. Speechlessness: causal attributions, emotional features and social consequences. J. Lang. Soc. Psychol. 23 (2), 147–179.

Betancourt, J.R., Corbett, J., Bondaryk, M.R., 2014. Addressing disparities and achieving equity: cultural competence, ethics, and health-care transformation. Chest. 145 (1), 143–148.

Bhat, B.V., Kingsley, M.K., 2020. Effective non-verbal communication Effective Medical Communication. Springer, Singapore, pp. 39–47.

Bonvillain, N., 2019. Language, Culture, and Communication: The Meaning of Messages. Rowman & Littlefield, Lanham.

Brooks, L.A., Manias, E., Bloomer, M.J., 2019. Culturally sensitive communication in healthcare: a concept analysis. Collegian. 26 (3), 383–391.

Cai, M., 2019. Reflection of Cultural Difference of the East and the West in Nonverbal Communication. 1st International Symposium on Education, Culture and Social Sciences (ECSS 2019). Advances in Social Science, Education and Humanities Research. Atlantis Press.

Carroll, J., Epstein, R., Fiscella, K., Gipson, T., Volpe, E., Jean-Pierre, P., 2007. Caring for Somali women: implications for clinician-patient communication. Patient Educ Couns. 66 (3), 337–345.

Cross, W.M., Bloomer, M.J., 2010. Extending boundaries: clinical communication with culturally and linguistically diverse mental health clients and carers. Int. J. Ment. Health Nurs. 19 (4), 268–277.

Crowther, S., Lau, A., 2019. Migrant polish women overcoming communication challenges in Scottish maternity services: a qualitative descriptive study. Midwifery. 72, 30–38.

De Maesschalck, S., Deveugele, M., Willems, S., 2011. Language, culture and emotions: exploring ethnic minority patients' emotional expressions in primary healthcare consultations. Patient Educ Couns. 84 (3), 406–412.

Douglas, M.K., Pierce, J.U., Rosenkoetter, M., Pacquiao, D., Callister, L.C., Hattar-Pollara, M., et al., 2013. Standards of practice for culturally competent nursing care: 2011 update. J. Transcult. Nurs. 22 (4), 317–333.

Dune, T., Perz, J., Mengesha, Z., Ayika, D., 2017. Culture Clash? Investigating constructions of sexual and reproductive health from the perspective of 1.5 generation migrants in Australia using Q methodology. Reprod. Health. 14 (1), 50.

El-Amouri, S., O'Neill, S., 2011. Supporting cross-cultural communication and culturally competent care in the linguistically and culturally diverse hospital settings of UAE. Contemp. Nurse. 39 (2), 240–255.

Elfenbein, H.A., Ambady, N., 2002. On the universality and cultural specificity of emotion recognition: a meta-analysis. Psychol. Bull. 128 (2), 203.

Estacio, E.V., Whittle, R., Protheroe, J., 2019. The digital divide: examining socio-demographic factors associated with health literacy, access and use of internet to seek health information. J. Health Psychol. 24 (12), 1668–1675.

Feldman, L.A., 1993. Distinguishing depression and anxiety in self-report: evidence from confirmatory factor analysis on nonclinical and clinical samples. J. Consult. Clin. Psychol. 61 (4), 631.

Floyd, S., Rossi, G., Baranova, J., Blythe, J., Dingemanse, M., Kendrick, K.H., et al., 2018. Universals and cultural diversity in the expression of gratitude. R. Soc. Open Sci. 5 (5), 180391.

Giger, J.N., Haddad, L., 2020. Transcultural Nursing-E-Book: Assessment and Intervention. Elsevier Health Sciences, Missouri.

Hua, Z., 2013. Exploring Intercultural Communication: Language in Action. Routledge, London, pp. 1–280.

Hull, R.H., 2016. The art of nonverbal communication in practice. Hear. J. 69 (5), 22–24.

Johnstone, M.J., Hutchinson, A.M., Redley, B., Rawson, H., 2016. Nursing roles and strategies in end-of-life decision making concerning elderly immigrants admitted to acute care hospitals: an Australian study. J. Transcult. Nurs. 27 (5), 471–479.

Jonkers, M., Richters, A., Zwart, J., 2011. Severe maternal morbidity among immigrant women in the Netherlands: patients' perspectives. Reprod. Health Matters 19 (37), 144–153.

Kee, J.W., Khoo, H.S., Lim, I., Koh, M.Y., 2018. Communication skills in patient-doctor interactions: learning from patient complaints. Health Prof. Educ. 4 (2), 97–106.

Keltner, D., Ekman, P., Gonzaga, G.C., Beer, J., 2003. Facial expression of emotion. In: Davidson, R.J., Scherer, K.R., Goldsmith, H.H. (Eds.), Handbook of Affective Sciences. Oxford University Press, Oxford, pp. 415–432.

Kirch, M.S., 1979. Non-verbal communication across cultures. Mod. Lang. J. 63 (8), 416–423.

Kubilius, K. 2019. Non-verbal communication: yes and no in Bulgaria. https://www.thoughtco.com/nodding-yes-and-no-in-bulgaria-1501211.

Levine, C.S., Ambady, N., 2013. The role of non-verbal behaviour in racial disparities in health care: implications and solutions. Med. Educ. 47 (9), 867–876.

Levine, R., 1997. A Geography of Time. Basic Books, New York, NY.

Levine, T.R., Asada, K.J.K., Park, H.S., 2006. The lying chicken and the gaze avoidant egg: eye contact, deception, and causal order. South. Commun. J. 71 (4), 401–411.

Li, C., Son, N., Abdulkerim, B.A., Jordan, C.A., Son, C.G.E., 2017. Overcoming communication barriers to healthcare for culturally and linguistically diverse patients. N. Am. J. Med. Sci. (Boston) 10 (3), 103–109.

Lim, N., 2016. Cultural differences in emotion: differences in emotional arousal level between the East and the West. Integr. Med. Res. 5 (2), 105–109.

Lorié, Á., Reinero, D.A., Phillips, M., Zhang, L., Riess, H., 2017. Culture and nonverbal expressions of empathy in clinical settings: a systematic review. Patient Educ. Couns. 100 (3), 411–424.

Maier-Lorentz, M.M., 2008. Transcultural nursing: its importance in nursing practice. J. Cult. Divers. 15 (1), 37–43.

Mandal, F.B., 2014. Nonverbal communication in humans. J. Hum. Behav. Soc. Environ. 24 (4), 417–421.

Matsumoto, D., Hwang, H.S., 2011. Evidence for training the ability to read microexpressions of emotion. Motiv. Emot. 35 (2), 181–191.

Matsumoto, D., Yoo, S.H., Hirayama, S., Petrova, G., 2005. Validation of an individual-level measure of display rules: The Display Rule Assessment Inventory (DRAI). Emotion. 5, 23–40. https://doi.org/10.1037/1528-3542.5.1.23.

Matteliano, M.A., Street, D., 2012. Nurse practitioners' contributions to cultural competence in primary care settings. J. Am. Acad. Nurse Pract. 24 (7), 425–435.

McCreaddie, M., Payne, M., 2014. Humour in health-care interactions: a risk worth taking. Health Expect. 17 (3), 332–344.

McHugh, C., 1992. Cultural barriers to communication. Hum. Commun. Stud. 20, 109–128.

McLaren, H.J., 2016. Silence as a power. Soc. Altern. 35 (1), 3.

Mehrabian, A., 1972. Nonverbal Communication. Transaction Publishers, Oxon.

Mengesha, Z.B., Perz, J., Dune, T., Ussher, J., 2018. Talking about sexual and reproductive health through interpreters: the experiences of health care professionals consulting refugee and migrant women. Sex. Reprod. Healthc. 16, 199–205.

Merry, L.A., Gagnon, A.J., Kalim, N., Bouris, S.S., 2011. Refugee claimant women and barriers to health and social services post-birth. Can. J. Public Health. 102 (4), 286–290.

Nakane, I., 2006. Silence and politeness in intercultural communication in university seminars. J. Pragmat. 38, 1811–1835.

NMC, 2018. Code of Professional Conduct. Read. The Nursing and Midwifery Council. Available at: https://www.nmc.org.uk/standards/code/.

O'Hagan, S., Manias, E., Elder, C., Pill, J., Woodward-Kron, R., McNamara, T., et al., 2014. What counts as effective communication in nursing? Evidence from nurse educators' and clinicians' feedback on nurse interactions with simulated patients. J. Adv. Nurs. 70 (6), 1344–1355. https://doi.org/10.1111/jan.12296.

Pant, B., 2016. Different Cultures See Deadlines Differently. Available at https://hbr.org/2016/05/different-cultures-see-deadlines-differently.

Papadopoulos, I., Shea, S., Taylor, G., Pezzella, A., Foley, L., 2016. Developing tools to promote culturally competent compassion, courage, and intercultural communication in healthcare. J. Compassionate Health Care 3 (1), 2.

Parums-Aug, D., 2015. Is There a Role for Humour in Medicine? If so, what is it? *Healthcare professionals.* Available at: https://healthcare-arena.co.uk/tag/healthcare-professionals/.

Paternotte, E., Scheele, F., Seeleman, C.M., Bank, L., Scherpbier, A.J., van Dulmen, S., 2016. Intercultural doctor-patient communication in daily outpatient care: relevant communication skills. Perspect. Med. Educ. 5 (5), 268–275.

Phillimore, J., 2016. Migrant maternity in an era of superdiversity: new migrants' access to, and experience of, antenatal care in the West Midlands, UK. Soc. Sci. Med. 148, 152–159.

Pogosyan, M., 2015. Emotion perception across cultures. Available at: https://www.psychologytoday.com/gb/blog/between-cultures/201610/emotion-perception-across-cultures.

Price, C., 2013. Effective communication in midwifery. Br. J. Midwifery. 21 (6) 454–454.

Protheroe, J., Estacio, E.V., Saidy-Khan, S., 2015. Patient information materials in general practices and promotion of health literacy: an observational study of their effectiveness. Br. J. Gen. Pract. 65 (632), e192–e197.

Purnell, L., 2018. Cross cultural communication: verbal and non-verbal communication, interpretation and translation. In: Douglas, M., Pacquiao, D., Purnell, L. (Eds.), Global Applications of Culturally Competent Health Care: Guidelines for Practice. Springer, Cham. https://doi.org/10.1007/978-3-319-69332-3_14.

Richters, J., Khoei, E.M., 2008. Concepts of sexuality and health among Iranian women in Australia. Aust. Fam. Physician. 37 (3), 190.

Riera, A., Ocasio, A., Tiyyagura, G., Krumeich, L., Ragins, K., Thomas, A., et al., 2015. Latino caregiver experiences with asthma health communication. Qual. Health Res. 25 (1), 16–26.

Russell, J.A., Pratt, G., 1980. A description of the affective quality attributed to environments. J. Pers. Soc. Psychol. 38 (2), 311.

Said, A.J., 2018. Revisiting the perception of silence in linguistics. J. Adv. Linguist. 9, 1471–1477.

Schuessler, J., 2018. Think You Always Say Thank You? Oh Please. Available at: https://www.nytimes.com/2018/05/22/arts/23thank-you.html.

Shahid, S., Finn, L.D., Thompson, S.C., 2009. Barriers to participation of Aboriginal people in cancer care: communication in the hospital setting. Med. J. Aust. 190 (10), 574–579.

Sorensen, K., Pelikan, J.M., Röthlin, F., Ganahl, K., Slonska, Z., Doyle, G., et al., 2015. Health literacy in Europe: comparative results of the European health literacy survey (HLS-EU). Eur. J. Public Health. 25 (6), 1053–1058.

Suarez, N.R.E., Urtecho, M., Jubran, S., Yeow, M.E., Wilson, M.E., Boehmer, K.R., et al., 2021. The roles of medical interpreters in intensive care unit communication: a qualitative study. Patient Educ. Couns. 104 (5), 1100–1108.

Tennant, K., Long, A., Toney-Butler, T.J., 2020. Active Listening. *StatPearls [Internet].*

Tiwari, R., 2020. Listening makes communication effective and complete. Juni Khyat: UGC Care Group I Listed Journal. 10 (6) Available at: http://junikhyatjournal.in/no_13_jun_20/70.pdf.

Tsai, J.L., 2007. Ideal affect: cultural causes and behavioral consequences. Perspect. Psychol. Sci. 2 (3), 242–259.

Turner, J.H., Stets, J.E., 2005. The Sociology of Emotions. Cambridge University Press, Cambridge.

van Dulmen, S., 2017. Listen: when words don't come easy. Patient Educ Couns. 100 (11), 1975–1978.

Wang, W.C., Lin, C.H., Chu, Y.C., 2011. Cultural diversity and information and communication impacts on language learning. International Education Studies. 4 (2), 111–115.

Wankhede, M.S., 2013. Language and culture communication: a sociolinguistic perspective. Confluence. 2250, 138X.

Ward, M., Kristiansen, M., Sørensen, K., 2019. Migrant health literacy in the European Union: a systematic literature review. Health Educ. J. 78 (1), 81–95.

Wilson, E., Chen, A.H., Grumbach, K., Wang, F., Fernandez, A., 2005. Effects of limited English proficiency and physician language on health care comprehension. J. Gen. Intern. Med. 20 (9), 800–806.

World Health Organization, 2018. WHO Recommendations on Intrapartum Care for a Positive Childbirth Experience. World Health Organization.

Yue, S.W.Z., 2005. Eastern and western cultural differences from the view of nonverbal communication–time, space and silence communicating different nonverbal messages. J. Anshan Nor. Univ. 5, 016.

CHAPTER 3

Transcultural Beliefs, Values and Religious Practices

INTRODUCTION

A key skill for a midwife is to have a broad understanding of cultural values and beliefs. In this chapter, you will be provided with an overview of cultural beliefs, values, rituals and norms and how they may relate to the woman's behaviour during pregnancy. Key theories around cultural values will be explored with an aim to highlight how these are shaped by the environment. The importance of religion and spirituality is explored and how they can impact on practices relating to health. A review of religious and spiritual beliefs will provide insight on the impact on pregnancy and childbirth. Health belief systems in different cultures will provide an understanding of influences on health seeking behaviour.

Cultural Beliefs, Values, Norms and Tradition

WHAT ARE BELIEFS?

It is important to start this section with an understanding of what is a belief. The social nature of human beings means that we naturally live in communities to thrive and survive. Being part of a community leads to a shared way and understanding of doing things, such as eating, sleeping and giving birth. Human behaviour is learnt, and from this behaviour, a shared meaning of life is derived. Beliefs are often formed to protect communities and are the principles or convictions that people hold to be true. The beliefs that embody the myths, values and ideologies of a group are usually invisible to those who hold them and often results in behaviour that is inherent and second nature. Beliefs shape behaviour and guide how people carry out tasks and activities and can change for an individual depending on their life experiences and the contact they have with society. If you think of women who have lived in different parts of the world, their contact with other people may influence or change their beliefs. Therefore, the environment is an important factor in shaping a woman's beliefs. This is where acculturation discussed in Chapter 1 is relevant.

What Are Cultural Beliefs?

Cultural beliefs are the standards and expectations generated by culture. Cultural beliefs are defined as 'a set of behavioural patterns related to thoughts, manners and actions, which members of society have shared and passed on to succeeding generations' (Hatah et al., 2015). For example, different cultural groups have diverse belief systems about health and healing compared to the Western biomedical medicine model (Vaughn et al., 2009). Cultural beliefs often protect individuals from harm or adverse outcomes, and you must understand this concept. During pregnancy, fear of the consequences of not heeding standards or behaving in a particular way may lead the woman to adopt specific behaviours. Hence, you may face the challenge of advising a woman about care in pregnancy that conflicts with her cultural beliefs. Cultural beliefs are communicated amongst individuals, and it is important to note that not all members of a group will conform to these beliefs. However, during pregnancy, in some cultures, the woman may most likely conform to group beliefs to avoid harming her baby.

Cultural Norms

Norms refer to behaviour and attitudes which are considered normal; they encourage reliable guides for day-to-day living. Norms can also be the shared expectations and rules that guide the behaviour of people within groups. Culture has been classified into material and non-material aspects. Whilst material culture refers to the visible, tactile objects manufactured, non-material culture comprises the norms and customs of people. Material culture is concrete and takes the form of artefacts and crafts, whilst non-material culture is abstract but has a pervasive influence on the lives of a particular culture. Beliefs about good and evil, together with norms and taboos, are all good examples of non-material culture (Idang, 2015). Cultural norms lend meaning to life and include practices such as marriage rules and lifestyle choices. You need to be aware of cultural norms, as they may impact on the woman's health-seeking behaviour. It may be difficult for a woman to heed the advice given in pregnancy if it conflicts with a cultural norm. Later on in this chapter, we will discuss some cultural norms and their impact on pregnancy.

TRADITION

The word tradition is from the Latin word 'traders' or 'traderer', meaning to hand over. Tradition, as defined by the Collins English Dictionary (2008), is the *'Handing down from generation to generation of customs and beliefs or customs and practices of long standing'*.

Tradition is linked with symbolic meaning and significance with origins from the past. It is the holding of practices from a previous time that can be lost through industrialisation, globalisation and marginalisation of specific cultural groups (Green, 1997). It is presumed that at least two transmissions over three generations are required for a practice, belief or object to be seen as tradition (Shils, 1981). The customs and beliefs that are passed between generations help to maintain culture. Some traditions may be unique to families, and individuals can create others. Traditions are also a way of providing a sense of belonging that brings individuals and communities together. They provide a way of demonstrating values and providing a sense of stability, predictability and order. Individuals do not need to be located in a particular place for a culture to be maintained. Culture is sustained by this handing down of information provided there is an individual to continue these practices. This is a significant point for midwives caring for migrant women, whether they are first or second generation (second generation are people born in the UK to parents who migrated from outside the UK). There is a likelihood that culture may still be maintained even in the diaspora.

Cultural Rituals

Rituals are a common feature of all known human societies (Brown, 2004) and could include unique gestures and words and use of certain objects, consumption of special foods, drinks and drugs, amongst other things. Rituals of social interactions could include phrases such as saying 'thank you' or 'sorry' and sending greeting cards. More significant rituals could include family traditions during holidays and celebrations such as Christmas and Easter or during Muslim festivals and Chinese New Year. Distinctive rituals are especially relevant to a community and help reinforce a sense of identity and continuity with the past. Rituals are affected by the changes communities undergo in modern societies because they depend so much on the broad participation of practitioners and others in the communities themselves (United Nations Educational, Scientific and Cultural Organization (UNESCO) 2020). Processes such as migration, individualisation, the general introduction of formal education, the growing influence of major world religions and other effects of globalisation have a particularly marked effect on these practices (UNESCO, 2020). If you live in a multicultural society, you may be aware of some rituals, particularly if they are relevant to pregnancy and childbirth. Acknowledgement of these practices and their importance to women and their families are part of cultural sensitivity. Often antenatal appointments or even a planned labour induction may cause conflicts if scheduled during an important ritual. Even the simple act of not observing phrases such as saying 'hello' or giving an appropriate introduction can concern some women.

There may be cultural rituals that are specific to men and some specific to women. Rituals may be undertaken by the woman with no scientific evidence but performed as a believed form of protection. Some initiation rituals contain harmful practices, and others, even under the perspectives of modern society, are deemed to be harmless (Schlegel and Barry, 2017). Having some knowledge of harmful practices that could affect a person's health is required for all health-care professionals.

A rite of passage is a ritual event performed in traditional societies that marks a person's transition from one social position to another. This includes birth, coming-of-age, marriage and death as well as initiation into groups such as fraternity organisations (Bell, 1997). Initiation rituals or puberty rites are ceremonies of the transition from childhood into the next stage, in most societies, an adolescent stage (Schlegel and Barry, 1980; Schief et al., 2018). For example, puberty rituals found mainly in Africa and Asia involving mutilation of the female genitalia, a harmful practice with a lifelong physical and psychological impact on the woman. On the other hand, the ritual of male circumcision is practised worldwide in Western, Eastern, African and Asian societies and is deemed harmless and culturally accepted.

A study on 184 societies around the globe by Schlegel and Barry (1980) found approximately 36% of the worldwide societies have initiation ceremonies for boys, while 46% of them hold puberty rituals for girls. This study demonstrates how widespread these rituals are and an important component of many cultures. The duration, character and content of each stage are culturally explicit (Schlegel and Barry, 2017), which means that they are governed by culture. Transition ceremonies pertinent only to a particular aspect of social life are also present, such as the Jewish bar (and now bat) mitzvah and Christian confirmation, which apply only to the religious sphere of life, as well as the Hindu *upanayana*, a ceremony of spiritual rebirth for young boys of the three upper *varnas* (caste categories): Brahmin, Kshatriya and Vaisya (Tyler, 1973). Awareness of these rituals is important, particularly pertaining to any that may affect the woman's health. In addition, an understanding of the significance of rituals equips the midwife to engage in sensitive discussions that may prevent harmful practices.

Point to Remember

One can see how any rituals or practices related to pregnancy, which may be harmful, need to be explored with the woman in order to gain some negotiation and compromise during pregnancy. The inability of the midwife to explore possible rituals with women prevents appropriate advice from being given.

What Are Values?

Values are termed as what is right and wrong and what is important in life (Idang, 2015). Every person has values, and how they practice this relies on various factors. Values are used to distinguish cultural groups, societies and individuals and to explain the motivational foundation of attitudes and behaviour (Schwartz, 2012). Values may also be structured similarly across culturally diverse groups; however, individuals and groups may differ and have different values, priorities or 'hierarchies (Schwartz, 2012). A value can be seen as some point of view or conviction which we can live with, live by and make ultimate sacrifices for (Idang, 2015). Therefore, if an individual wishes to maintain their values, this can create stress when they are not achievable. The fact that a woman's values are influenced by many factors that affect all aspects of her life is an important note for midwives. Values permeate every aspect of human life, which could be religious, political, social, moral and cultural (Idang, 2015). In some instances, a woman may have a personal value that is not influenced by any external forces. The significance of values influenced by cultural factors should be noted by the midwife, as these may be controlled by the family, community, political and societal environment.

As already suggested, women in a society may have personal values, but they may also share collective values. It is interesting to note that although values often suggest how people should behave, they do not accurately reflect how people actually behave. Such is the essence of human nature to have these values, but in reality, adherence to these does depend on circumstances. For example, a person may have a value that telling untruths is not permitted; however, they may support telling untruths in certain situations. The importance of values is that they define what people care about and are revealed by their priorities and influence every aspect of their lives. In the next section, we will look at the specific features of values and how they are connected and motivated.

Schwartz's Theory of Basic Human Values

Schwartz's (2012) theory of basic human values states features that are common to all values and what distinguishes one value from another is the type of goal or motivation that it expresses.

Schwartz (2012) states that values are likely to be grounded in one or more requirements of human existence, which are needs as individuals as biological organisms, requisites of coordinated social interaction and survival and welfare needs of groups. It is suggested that humans cannot cope with the requirements of human existence on their own and need to communicate with others and gain cooperation. Schwartz's (2012) results from several studies of more than 25,000 people in 44 countries with wide-ranging cultures suggested that there are 56 specific universal values that are stated to be the same worth for almost all people. The Schwartz (2012) theory of basic values is identified in 10 broad personal values which are recognised across cultures and are distinguished by four dimensions of underlying goals or motivation: openness to change, self-enhancement, conservation and self transcendence. Under each dimension, 10 basic values identified by Schwartz (2012) are presented (see Fig. 3.1).

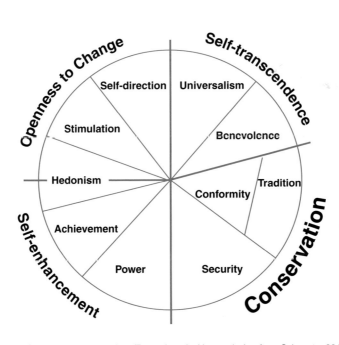

Fig. 3.1 Schwartz's human value. (Reproduced with permission from Schwartz, 2012.)

Openness to change is said to be motivated by self-direction, stimulation and hedonism.

1. **Self-direction** derives from people's need for control, autonomy and independence. The goal of this value is independent thought and action in choosing, creating and exploring.
2. **Stimulation** derives from the need for variety and stimulation to achieve excitement, novelty and be positive to face challenges in life.
3. **Hedonism** derives from the need to enjoy life, pleasure or painless gratification for oneself. Happiness is not included because people achieve it through attaining whatever outcomes they value.

Self-enhancement is said to be motivated by achievement and power.

4. **Achievement** emphasises personal success through demonstrating competence according to social standards.
5. **Power** is social status and prestige, control or dominance over people and resources. Sample of power: Authority, wealth and social power.

Conservation is said to be motivated by security, conformity and tradition

6. **Security**: Safety, harmony and stability of society, of relationships and self. Sample of security action: social order and safety.
7. **Conformity**: Restraint of everyday actions (mostly within-group or closed ones), inclinations and impulses likely to upset or harm others and violate social expectations or norms. Sample of conformity action: obedient, self-discipline, politeness and filial piety.
8. **Tradition:** Values demand responsiveness to expectations from the past, which include respect, commitment and acceptance of the customs and ideas that one's culture or religion provides. Tradition and conformity values are especially close motivationally, as they share imposed expectations from society.

Self-transcendence is said to be motivated by benevolence and universalism.

9. **Benevolence**: Preserving and enhancing the welfare of those with whom one is in frequent personal contact. Benevolence values accentuate voluntarily acts for other's welfare—sample of benevolence: helpful, honest and loyal.
10. **Universalism**: Understanding, appreciation, tolerance and protection for the welfare of all people and nature. The universalism values derive from the survival needs of an individual and groups. However, people do not recognise these needs until their life is threatened, or they become aware of the scarcity of natural resources.

The focus of Schwartz's (2012) theory is that values form a circular structure (see Fig. 3.1) that reflect the motivation that each value conveys. Relations among these 10 broad personal values are fluid. For example, a woman attempting to pursue one action may face consequences that conflict with some values but are compatible with others. The values of benevolence and power conflict with each other, while conformity and security are compatible. The practical, psychological, and social consequences of not following values should not be overlooked. It is possible for a woman to adhere to competing values, but this is not usually done in a single act (Schwartz, 2012), and of course, people can and do pursue competing values. A woman may do so through different acts, at different times and in different settings. In the next section, we will look at some suggested broad themes of cultural values and how these can be related to women during pregnancy.

What Are Cultural Values?

It is suggested that at the centre of culture is a system of societal norms consisting of the value systems (or the mental software) shared by major groups in a population (Gaygısız et al., 2017), highlighting that values are an essential part of national culture and are shared by the majority. It is interesting to note that values portray an ideal culture and the standards society would like to embrace and live up to. Therefore, individuals who want to remain inclusive in a family, community or society may adopt these cultural values. A person may be taught these values at an early age, usually by their parents, but values can also be taught in an educational or organisational environment. A person's values are not static; they vary across time and between groups, as people change their views and societal beliefs. Values may also vary from culture to culture, but the assumption should not be made that a person from the same culture has the same values. Cultural change has occurred over the centuries as a result of influences such as Western-style education, globalisation, rural-urban migration and the introduction of Christianity. Yet, many central values (e.g., kinship systems and ties, the importance of spirituality, honouring elders, expectations in romantic relationships) persist (Goodwin et al., 2012; Darkwah, 2016).

Hofstede's Cultural Values

According to Hofstede et al. (2010), cultural values are our reactions to the environment we live in, and we are taught those values at a young age. Values are a culture's standard for discerning what is good and just in society and can be deeply ingrained and are significant for teaching a culture's beliefs. Hofstede (2010) proposed that culture is composed of six empirically identified dimensions:

- Power distance (inequality between people),
- Individualism vs. collectivism (the integration of individuals into primary groups),
- Masculinity vs. femininity (the division of emotional roles between males and females)
- Uncertainty avoidance (the level of stress in a society related to unknown future),
- Short-term orientation and long-term orientation,
- Indulgence vs. restraint dimensions (Hofstede, 2010).

According to Hosftede's research of over 50 countries, there may be the adoption of particular values at the national level, which were infiltrated down to organisations, communities, families and even the individual (Hofstede, 2010). Certain countries were said to score high with particular dimensions. This highlights an interesting point on how society and national culture can conform to particular values. However, care should be taken not to stereotype due to the wide range of individuals within each national culture. Table 3.1 (Hofstede, 1991), gives examples of which countries scored high in each dimension.

Power Distance

If you look at (Hofstede, 2010), the cultural dimension model, societies that have high power distance values may result in women lacking control in their health-seeking behaviour. It is stated that all societies are unequal, but it is important to note that some are more unequal than others (Hofstede, 2011). Consequently, a society's values may reflect this. For example, in low power distance societies, parents may treat children as equals and inequalities are minimised; whereas in high power societies, children are expected to be obedient to parents and inequalities are expected and desired. Hofstede (2011) states that in high power distance societies, these are cultures in which the power relations are paternalistic, subordinates expect to be told what to do and older people are respected and often feared. A woman who lives in a society that mainly conforms to high power distance values may face a lack of choice in her health-seeking behaviour and may be influenced by authoritarian figures such as healthcare professionals. The opposite is found in lower power societies where the use of power should be legitimate, subordinates expect to be consulted and older people are neither respected nor feared (Hofstede, 2011). Hence, women who have lived in lower power societies may be used to more freedom in making choices about their health and would not automatically deem that anyone that offers advice in a position of authority should be heeded.

TABLE 3.1 ▪ Hofstede's Cultural Dimension Model

Cultural Dimension	Definition	Examples
Power distance	**Power distance** is the extent to which the less powerful members of institutions and organisations within a country expect and accept that power is distributed unequally.	**Low:** US and Canada **High:** Japan and Singapore
Individualism and collectivism	**Individualism** describes cultures in which the ties between individuals are loose. **Collectivism** describes cultures in which people are integrated into strong, cohesive groups that protect individuals in exchange for unquestioning loyalty.	**Individualistic:** US, Australia and Great Britain **Collectivistic:** Singapore, Hong Kong and Mexico
Masculinity-femininity	**Masculinity** pertains to cultures in which social gender roles are clearly distinct. **Femininity** describes cultures in which social gender roles overlap.	**Masculinity:** Japan, Austria and Italy **Femininity:** Sweden, Norway and Netherlands
Uncertainty avoidance (UAI)	**Uncertainty avoidance** is the extent to which the members of a culture feel threatened by uncertain or unknown situations.	**Low:** Singapore, Jamaica and Denmark **High:** Greece, Portugal and Japan
Confucian dynamism	**Confucian dynamism** denotes the time orientation of a culture, defined as a continuum with long-term and short-term orientations as its two poles.	**Long-term:** China and Japan **Short-term:** US and Canada

Reproduced with permission from Hofstede, G., 1991. Cultures and Organizations: Software of the Mind. Berkshire, England: McGraw-Hill Book Company Europe.

Individualistic Versus Collective Societies

In individualistic societies, the ties between individuals are loose; everyone is expected to look after themselves and their immediate family, whereas in collective societies, individuals are born into groups or communities which are cohesive and protective (Hofstede et al., 2010). Women are expected to be independent in individualistic societies; matters concerning health are very much kept within the family unit. In collective societies, people from birth onwards are integrated into strong, cohesive in-groups, often extended families (with uncles, aunts and grandparents) that provide protection in exchange for loyalty (Hofstede, 2011). Women may rely more on the family and community for advice, including matters concerning health. Transgression of any values may not lead to guilt in individual societies as opposed to guilt in collective societies. According to Hofstede et al. (2010), individualism tends to be dominant in developed and Western countries and collectivism in less developed and Eastern countries.

Masculinity Versus Feminist Societies

Masculinity versus its opposite, femininity, as a societal, not as an individual characteristic, refers to the distribution of values between genders (Hofstede, 2011). In masculine societies, gender roles are clearly distinct – men are expected to be assertive and deal with facts; in feminine societies, both men and women are supposed to be modest (Hofstede et al., 2010). In feminine societies, women are more likely to decide on the number of children, not men. This is an important consideration during pregnancy when decisions are made by both men and women in some societies equally or by men alone. Taboos are based on deeply rooted values, and in masculine societies, even though women may be as assertive as men, there are still gaps between men's values and women's values (Hofstede, 2011).

High Uncertainty Versus Low Uncertainty Societies

In the case of societies that demonstrate high uncertainty avoidance, there is an increased awareness of being threatened by ambiguous or unknown situations (Hofstede et al., 2010). For example, anything that is unusual is considered dangerous in high uncertainty avoidance societies, as opposed to a subject of curiosity in low uncertainty avoidance societies. High uncertainty avoiding cultures try to minimise the possibility of unusual or new situations using strict behavioural codes, laws and rules and disapproval of deviant opinions (Hofstede, 2011). Individuals from high uncertainty avoidance countries are said to be more emotional, while low uncertainty avoidance cultures are more tolerant of different opinions, have fewer rules and are not likely to express emotion. Having some insight into a woman's values is important for a midwife, particularly around how she may make any decisions about the care she receives during pregnancy. It is important to have discussions with women to understand the values that are important in her culture and why they may adhere to these. In this way, midwives can avoid inadvertently being culturally insensitive to the woman's worldview and protect her cultural identity.

Short Versus Long-Term Orientation Societies

Societies with short-term orientation are normative societies that prefer to maintain traditions and view societal change with suspicion. Societies scoring high on long-term orientation are, on the other hand, more pragmatic and oriented towards future rewards, in particular saving, persistence and adapting to changing circumstances (Hofstede, 2010). Women who value short-term orientation are more likely to be focused on the present or the past and may have little concern about future events. In contrast, women who have long-term orientation perspectives may be more focused on future events and less likely to adhere to traditions and social norms in the present.

In following Hofstede's (2010) cultural values, care must be taken to avoid expecting women to behave in a particular way due to their background. Women may just as easily not conform to a country's values and may indeed not follow any cultural value. However, this knowledge can increase midwives' awareness of how women's values can be very different from their own. Remember, cultural awareness is about being aware of how your cultural values may differ from that of the woman you are caring for. It is the recognition of this that provides insight into the woman's perspective.

Exercise

After reading Schwartz's and Hofstede's cultural values, please read the following scenario and think about the values that Elsa may be adhering to in this situation.

Elsa has concerns about how her antenatal care has been scheduled. Elsa has tried several times to discuss her antenatal care with the midwife but has felt unable to challenge the care provided to her. It is not usual for Elsa to question other people who are in an authority position. She is unable to voice this concern to the midwife.

Learning Activity

Take a moment to think of any cultural beliefs or values you may have. Where did they originate? How did you learn of these beliefs and values, and why have you continued to follow them? Consider any rituals that you perform. Why are these rituals important to you? If you were unable to perform these rituals, what impact would this have on you?

Religion and Spirituality

Midwives should be aware of the role and impact of spiritual and religious beliefs on the woman's life and on her health-seeking behaviour. The two terms are used interchangeably; however, spirituality and religiosity are separate but related concepts. Spirituality denotes an inner freedom to engage in faith and a relationship with a Supreme Being, such as God, whereas religion refers to the outward commitment to highly prescribed beliefs, practices and rituals related to the Supreme Being, such as church attendance and associated activities (Greer and Abel, 2017). Another way to distinguish between the two terms is that religion has theological beliefs and practices with commitments and congregational activities, whereas spirituality has more focus on the individual and might not have an association with an organised institution (Plante and Sherman, 2001).

Spirituality is generally experienced and expressed individually, and the level of depth or intensity of spirituality differs from person to person (Lepherd, 2015). Differences can be due to ethnicity, culture and the environment the person lives in. Even if individuals share the same culture, their spirituality may be different and persons from different religions will experience different spirituality; for instance, the spirituality of a Christian may be different from that of a Hindu. Spirituality is also regarded as a universal human phenomenon, and it is present in everyone whether they practice a religion or not (Goddard, 1995). This is an important factor in responding to people who state that they are not spiritual just because they are not religious. The significance here is that no single faith or religious tradition can claim that their understanding of spirituality is unique to a specific way of thinking, but rather it is a characteristic of humanity (Lepherd, 2015). In midwifery, recognising the woman's spirituality is a crucial component of care and should not be relegated to the background (Crowther and Hall, 2015; Lewinson et al., 2015). Spirituality for some women is a way of coping with changes in lifestyle and stressors that can be caused by pregnancy. Often, this spirituality provides the woman with the ability to overcome challenges caused by the choices that she must make about her pregnancy.

In many cases, culture and religion are not so distinct, with cultural practices becoming 'religionised', and religious ideas becoming part of a culture (Abdulla, 2018). While it is suggested that religion affects cultures (Beckford and Demerath, 2007), religion itself is also affected by culture and is an essential layer of culture. Often the line between what is a cultural practice and religious practice becomes blurred. Therefore, it imports that when studying religion, a study of culture is necessary. This statement is argued from three positions by Beyers (2017), who highlights that:

- Cultural migrations are occurring worldwide.
- Religion as a cultural identity marker causes the borders between culture and religion to blur.
- The location of religion within culture causes religion to act as custodian of culture (Beyers, 2017).

Due to migration, which has increased greatly in the last 50 years, culture has crossed borders and maintenance of practices has been maintained by religion. It is also difficult to study religion without studying ethnicity, and understanding the nature of religion can only be achieved when one understands its connection to ethnicity and culture (Beyers, 2017). The difficulty for midwives is understanding what is a cultural practice as opposed to religious practice. In some instances, it is better to take any practices, whatever their origin, as of equal significance. It should not be the midwife's role to argue for one or the other but to accept the woman's viewpoint. For example, Ramadan (2010) maintains that Islam must not be viewed as a culture; it is argued that the two are very distinct, with a clear purpose for each. The essence of Islam is stated to be religious, not cultural (Ramadan, 2010). Many adherents of different religions will agree to this when applied to their own religious convictions (Beyers, 2017). There are also other arguments that some religions can be thought of as cultures (e.g., Judaism is a culture) (Cohen and Varnum, 2016), as the practices of Judaism are cultural.

The study of religion is difficult when the borders of religion and other identifying elements overlap. There seem to be three scenarios to this problem (MacKay, 2000):

1. The ethnicity of a group is explained in terms of their religious beliefs. An example would be Jewish ethnicity, as it is the result of practising Judaism. Religion is the primary element in Jewish identity.
2. Religion is explained as the result of ethnicity. Muslim belief is the result of Arab ethnicity. The group's ethnic identity is the primary element in determining identity.
3. More elements than religion and ethnicity are at play in determining group identity. Elements such as language, geography, values, worldview and a shared history are examples.

Religion is naturally displayed, using symbolism, places of worship and sermons (Abdulla, 2018), whereas culture is not easily visible or seen, as discussed in Chapter 1. A significant note for midwives is in understanding that women often turn to their religious and spiritual beliefs when making decisions about their pregnancy. Religion and spirituality can impact decisions regarding diet, medicines based on animal products, modesty, strict prayer times that may interfere with medical treatment and the preferred gender of healthcare professionals (Swihart et al., 2021). Religion should be recognised in healthcare as source of personal strength which can be utilised during ill health (Hordern, 2016). Midwives should seek to know women's religious affiliation as part of the provision of holistic care. The Department of Health (DOH) for England and the Royal College of Psychiatrists emphasise the potential value of spirituality and prayer to patients' mental health and well-being (DOH, 2009). Moreover, the DOH asserts that 'an individual's religion or beliefs are increasingly acknowledged as playing an important role in the overall healing process' (DOH, 2009), emphasising that midwives should value the positive impact of religious beliefs on women's health.

OVERVIEW OF MAIN RELIGIONS

There are more than 4000 different religions and faiths in the entire world; three major religions are Islam, Christianity and Judaism (Yen, 2020). These religions have numerous sects and denominations that practice an individual set of beliefs with one singular god or deity. In addition, other religions that midwives may come in contact with are Hinduism and Buddhism, as well as African traditional religions. Culturally competent healthcare professionals recognise that there are differences and similarities within and between these religions (Wehbe-Alamah et al., 2020). Midwives who have increased their knowledge in the main religions are able to understand the importance to the woman of observing her religion during pregnancy and childbirth.

CHRISTIANITY

The term *Christian* is used to refer to a believer in Christianity. It has become the largest of the world's religions and, geographically, the most widely diffused of all faiths. The largest Christian groups are the Roman Catholic Church, the Eastern Orthodox churches and the Protestant churches (Stefon, 2020). The holy book of Christianity is the Bible, and tenets of Christianity are stated in the Apostles' Creed, which states that God created the earth, that Jesus Christ the Son of God was conceived by the Holy Spirit and was born of the virgin Mary. Christians believe in the Holy Spirit and the church, the forgiveness of sins, the communion of saints (living and dead), the resurrection of the body and eternal life (Erwin et al., 2017). As a tradition, Christianity is more than a system of religious beliefs but is said to have generated a culture, a set of ideas and ways of life, practices and artefacts that have been handed down from generation to generation since Jesus first became the object of faith (Stefon, 2020). The holy days of Christianity are Christmas (the birth of Jesus), Good Friday (the day Jesus was crucified) and Easter, the most important day, believed to be the day Jesus rose from the dead.

Roman Catholics account for the largest Christian church in the world, mainly in Latin America and Europe. The Catholic Church is led by the Pope, who resides in Vatican City. The Catholic Church is guided by the Holy Spirit, who in turn guides the Pope. Similar to other Christians, followers of the Catholic faith believe Jesus is a divine person, the Son of God, and that he died so that his people could live forever in heaven. The Catholic Church celebrates seven sacraments (a religious ceremony or ritual regarded as imparting divine grace). These sacraments are Baptism, Confirmation (affirms Christian belief and admission as a full member of the Church), Eucharist (celebration of the last supper of Jesus), Confession (repairing one's relationship with God), Anointing of the sick, Holy orders (being ordained as a priest, deacon or Bishop) and Holy Matrimony (Marriage). These rituals are important components of Roman Catholic practices.

The Eastern Orthodox church has followers in Eastern Europe, Greece, southwestern Asia, Georgia, Armenia, Azerbaijan and southeastern Russia. The Eastern Orthodox church believes in the birth of Jesus, the incarnation and resurrection. However, the Holy Spirit is seen as the guide to the church, operating through priests and bishops. The seven sacraments are also practised by the Orthodox church. However, the church is not led by the Pope but is governed by Bishops. The Orthodox Church celebrates religious festivals on different dates to Catholics and Protestants. For example, Christmas Day, celebrated by Catholics and Protestants on December 25, is marked by Orthodox Christians around January 7.

Pentecostalism is a protestant Christian movement that believes that all Christians can attain a direct personal experience of God through baptism with the Holy Spirit. Pentecostals also have the belief that faith is experiential and not achieved by rituals. There is no hierarchical structure in Pentecostalism, such as the Pope in Catholicism. In Western societies, Pentecostalism is strong in black churches in the UK, America, Australia and Asia. Baptism with the Holy Spirit is also believed to be accompanied by a sign, the gift of tongues. This 'speaking in tongues' occurs as speech in an unknown language or speech in a language known to others but not the speaker. The primary belief of classical Pentecostalism is that sins can be forgiven through death, burial and the resurrection of Jesus Christ.

The Church of England, another protestant denomination, is the primary church of England which states that the Bible is the principal foundation of all Christian faith. Followers perform the sacraments of baptism and holy communion, and like Pentecostalism, the Pope is not recognised. The Seventh-day Adventist Church is also a protestant denomination which is different due to the observance of Saturday being the seventh day and a holy day as opposed to Sunday. Followers of this movement are mainly situated in the US, where it was founded. However, followers are found all over the world. Most of the beliefs of Seventh-Day Adventists are similar to that of mainstream Christian churches. The church is known for its emphasis on diet and health and holistic understanding of the person (Sábaté et al., 2016).

Jehovah's Witnesses view themselves as Christian and regard Jesus Christ as the Son of God but not in the sense of being equal with God or one with God. Jehovah's Witnesses consider their religion to be a restoration of original first-century Christianity. They accept both the Old and New Testaments of the Bible as inspired by God. They do not, however, use the symbol of the cross because they believe it to be of pagan origin. The Jehovah's Witnesses deny the immortality of the soul, the existence of hell, and the seven sacraments. However, they do have a ritual of baptism. There is no observance of holy days, such as Christmas and Easter–except the Memorial of the Last Supper, which they hold once a year. Jehovah's Witnesses have religious beliefs that do not permit the transfusion of blood products and the use of some medical procedures (Chae et al., 2021).

Many Christians simply engage in eating a healthy and balanced diet. Other Christians may have more specific dietary needs and restrictions, such as Eastern Orthodox Christians who participate in fasting and abstaining as a spiritual practice (Alexiou, 2016). Seventh-Day

Adventists usually adhere to a healthy vegetarian diet and may also undertake fasting (Sábaté et al., 2016). The wide variety of dietary practices among Christians means that midwives are required to discuss them with each woman who identifies as Christian as to what their dietary needs are.

JUDAISM

The term *Jewish* is used to refer to a religion, culture or people (Purnell, 2014). Jews vary in their approach to Jewish traditions, laws and ritual observance; the major religious streams of Judaism are Reformed, Conservative, Orthodox and Reconstructionist. Many Jews do not identify with any one denomination, instead describing themselves as 'nondenominational' or 'just Jewish'. The Torah, the foundation document of Judaism, includes 613 commandments of detailed instructions on principles of how to live. There are 13 principles of the Jewish faith (see Table 3.2). These principles are usually recited during congregations every day after morning prayers in the synagogue.

Shabbat (the Sabbath) is the most important time of the week for Jews. It begins on Friday evenings and ends at sunset on Saturdays. During Shabbat, Jews remember that God created the world, and on the seventh day, he rested; hence, the belief that God's day of rest was a Saturday. Observing Shabbat can take many forms, depending on the type of Judaism that a Jewish family may follow. Orthodox and Conservative Jews, for example, may refrain from performing any physical labour, using any electrical device or other prohibited activities. Jewish holy days include the Passover festival, which retells the story of Israelites fleeing Egypt, Rosh Hashanah, which is Jewish New Year's Day and Yom Kippur, the day of atonement when people fast and pray.

Strict rules of *kashrut* (kosher) are typically observed by Jewish individuals who identify themselves as Orthodox. *Shechita* refers to the slaughtering of animals and includes no interruption of the incision, no tearing of tissues or covering the blood with earth and requires the removal of blood and forbidden fat (Tieman and Hassan, 2015). Kosher meat must come from an animal that has a cloven hoof and chews the cud to be regarded as clean (Popovsky, 2010). In addition, milk and meat should not be served together, and all pork products, including gelatine, are forbidden. Women who observe Orthodox Judaism may request either kosher or vegetarian meals when hospitalised.

TABLE 3.2 ■ **Thirteen Principles of the Jewish Faith**

1. Belief in the existence of the Creator, who is perfect in every manner of existence and is the primary cause of all that exists
2. The belief in God's absolute and unparalleled unity
3. The belief in God's non-corporeality, nor that He will be affected by any physical occurrences, such as movement, or rest or dwelling
4. The belief in God's eternity
5. The imperative to worship God exclusively and no foreign false gods
6. The belief that God communicates with man through prophecy
7. The belief in the primacy of the prophecy of Moses our teacher
8. The belief in the divine origin of the Torah
9. The belief in the immutability (unchangeable) of the Torah
10. The belief in God's omniscience and providence
11. The belief in divine reward and retribution
12. The belief in the arrival of the Messiah and the messianic era
13. The belief in the resurrection of the dead

Reproduced with permission from Chabad.org (2005). The Thirteen Principles of Jewish Faith. Available at: https://www.chabad.org/library/article_cdo/aid/332555/jewish/Maimonides-13-Principles-of-Faith.htm.

ISLAM

Islam is the main religion of the Middle East, North Africa and Asia. There are many denominations in Islam, with the two major ones being Sunni (85%) and Shia (or Shiite) (Arthington, 2019). In Arabic, Islam means 'surrender' to the will of Allah (Arabic name for God). Adherents to Islam referred to as Muslims, submit to the will of Allah (Rassool, 2014). The primary source of Islamic teachings is the *Koran* (the holy book for Muslims), followed by the *Sunnah* (deeds, practices and examples of Prophet Muhammad). Muslims believe in the Six Articles of Faith and the Five Pillars of Islam, core beliefs that shape Muslim thought, deed and society (see Table 3.3). It is believed that a Muslim who fulfils the five pillars of Islam remains in the faith and relents their sins will make it to Jannah (paradise).

TABLE 3.3 ■ Five Pillars of Islam and Six Articles of faith

Shahada *(Faith)* The declaration of faith in one God (Allah) and his messenger (peace be upon him)	The belief in Muhammad as the last messenger of God is the central tenet of Islam around which everything else revolves, and reciting the **Shahada** in prayer each day serves to remind Muslims of this integral belief
Salah *(Prayer)* The ritual prayer required of every Muslim five times a day throughout their lifetime	**Salah** *(salat)* occurs five times a day, and offers five different opportunities for remembrance of Allah and the purpose in this life to worship him
Sawm *(Fasting)* The act of fasting during the holy month of Ramadan	The month of Ramadan requires every Muslim to abstain from their most basic needs and desires, like food, drink and sexual relations for a period of time each day. Each year the **Sawm** gives Muslims the opportunity to gather control over their human needs. Without these distractions, Muslims can instead nurture good conduct and their connection to Allah
Zakat *(Almsgiving)* The act of giving a portion of a Muslim's wealth to those in need throughout their lifetime	It is obligatory to offer **Zakat** (alms) once a year, ensuring that wealth is continuously redistributed to those who are in need of it
Hajj *(Pilgrimage)* The sacred pilgrimage to Mecca required of every Muslim at least once in their lifetime if it is within their means	During the **Hajj** (pilgrimage), Muslims must each wear the same simple garments and perform the same ritual acts of devotion to Allah. Stripped of worldly distinction, people are reminded that all are equal before God

Six Articles of Faith:
1. **Allah:** the existence of one God, who alone created and sustains the universe
2. **Angels:** messengers of Allah who can communicate with humanity
3. **Holy Books:** the scriptures, including the Qur'an but also elements of the Tanakh (Hebrew Bible) and the message preached by Isa (Jesus)
4. **Prophets:** the messengers and prophets of Allah who came before Muhammad
5. **Day of Judgement:** a day on which Allah will assess the character of each person and either send them to heaven or hell
6. **Predestination:** Allah knows everything that will happen, although the common view is that humans still have free will to make choices

From 5 Pillars of Islam - What are the five pillars? | Islamic relief UK. Available at: https://www.islamic-relief.org.uk/islamic-resources/5-pillars-of-islam/.
From Six articles of faith. Understanding religion: An OCRS project. Available at: https://www.understandingreligion.org.uk/p/six-articles/.

The basic principle in Islam is that all foods created by Allah are permitted, with a few exceptions that are prohibited. This includes pork, blood, the meat of animals that died of causes other than proper slaughtering, food that has been dedicated or sacrificed to someone other than Allah, alcohol, intoxicants and inappropriately used drugs (Regenstein et al., 2003). Foods containing ingredients such as gelatine, enzymes, emulsifiers and flavours are questionable because the origin of these ingredients is not known. In the meat and poultry food industry, animals such as cows, veal, lamb, sheep, goats, turkeys, chickens, ducks, game birds, bison, venison, etc., are considered halal, but they must be prepared according to Islamic laws for their meat to be suitable for consumption. Halal is an Arabic word meaning 'lawful' or 'permitted'; in reference to food, it is the dietary standard, as prescribed in the Koran. The opposite of halal is haram, which means 'unlawful' or 'prohibited'. Halal and haram are universal terms that apply to all facets of a Muslim's life. These terms are commonly used in relation to food products, meat products, cosmetics, personal care products, pharmaceuticals, food ingredients and food contact materials. Traditional halal meat is killed by hand and must be blessed by the slaughterman. Islam has strict laws on the proper method of slaughtering an animal. One, called dhabihah, requires a swift, deep incision with a sharp knife on the neck that cuts the jugular vein. For meat to be considered halal, the animal must be alive and healthy before it is killed, and all the blood must be drained from the body. In addition, fasting for religious reasons, such as during Ramadan in Islam, is common, and although pregnancy is exempt, this practice is still adhered to by women. This can have a negative impact on the pregnancy; for instance, a study conducted among pregnant Muslim women in the Netherlands revealed that women's adherence to Ramadan fasting during early pregnancy could lead to lower birth weight of newborns (Savitri et al., 2014).

AFRICAN TRADITIONAL RELIGIONS

African traditional religion, wherever it is practised, has some defining characteristics. For instance, it possesses the concept of a Supreme Being, which is invisible and indigenous. It holds a belief in the existence of the human soul, and the soul does not die with the body. African traditional religion also has the belief that good and bad spirits do exist and that communication with the Supreme Being is possible. Above all, African traditional religions hold a moral sense of justice and truth and the knowledge of the existence of good and evil (Umoh, 2005). African religious values seem to permeate every facet of the life of the African, and an African believes that anything can be instilled with spiritual significance (Idang, 2015).

HINDUISM

Hinduism is one of the oldest world religions dating back to around 1500 BC. Scriptures were originally written in Sanskrit, a language in which most Hindus of today are no longer literate, and therefore customs over the years have tended to be passed on by word of mouth (Gatrad et al., 2004). Hindus believe in a 'transcendent' God who may be worshipped in a variety of ways through different symbolic manifestations (for example, statues). There are three supreme Hindu Gods forming the Hindu Trinity (Sharma, 2000), Brahma (The Creator), Vishnu (The Preserver) and Shiva (The Destroyer). In the UK, the majority of Hindus are Vishnuvites (Lipner, 2004), meaning that they worship Vishnu. Many Hindus believe that a person is born into a caste or acquires it by behaviour. There are broadly four main castes: Brahmins (highest), Ksatriya (ruling caste), Vaisya (farmers and merchants) and Sudras (the untouchables); this latter group historically worked as servants in India (Gatrad et al., 2004). The caste system still has a stronghold on Hindu families, and the impact of this on customs (including birth) also extends to those who have migrated (Gatrad et al., 2004). Most Hindus are strict vegetarians and vegans; the consumption of fish/eggs/animal fats is not permitted in any form; this is also the case for supplements and vitamins.

BUDDHISM

Buddhism is a faith that was founded more than 2500 years ago in India. Its practice is most prominent in East and Southeast Asia, but its influence is growing in the West. Followers of Buddhism do not recognise a supreme god or deity but focus on achieving enlightenment—a state of inner peace and wisdom. The path to enlightenment is through the practice and development of morality, meditation and wisdom. The basic tenet of Buddhism includes the 'Four Noble Truths': existence is suffering *(dukkha)*; suffering has a cause, namely craving and attachment *(trishna)*; there is a cessation of suffering, which is nirvana (Harvey, 2013). Buddhism believes there is an eightfold path to the cessation of suffering, which are of right views, right resolve, right speech, right action, right livelihood, right effort, right mindfulness and right concentration (Emmanuel, 2013).

Exercise

A midwife is booking a woman and discusses her plan for a schedule of antenatal care.
    The woman explains that she would be unable to attend the next appointment as it will conflict with a religious holiday.
    1. What steps do you think the midwife should take to understand the woman's concern?
    2. Why do you think it is important that a woman's religious practices should be considered during pregnancy.
    3. In your practice, can you think of any instances where a similar issue has arisen?

Religion and Health

CHRISTIANITY AND HEALTH BELIEFS

Christians recognise suffering as a part of the life of Jesus and as part of human life, and they regard suffering in illness as valuable to themselves as an act of spiritually carrying the cross. The New Testament supports health, wellness and caregiving in the following ways: (a) Jesus facilitated spiritual and physical healing, (b) the physical body is regarded as important and (c) physical and spiritual healing are important missions of the church (Rush and Aboul-Enein, 2016).

One of the main issues with pregnant women who are Christian are those who are Jehovah's Witnesses. Women who practice this faith do not accept transfusion of blood or its major components (Kitahara et al., 2019). This is based on the belief that to be transfused with blood is equivalent to eating it, and therefore prohibited by scripture (Genesis 9, 4: Leviticus 17, 12: Acts 15, 29) (Marsh and Bevan, 2002). Jehovah's Witnesses' religious principles do not absolutely prohibit the use of minor blood components such as albumin, immune globulins and haemophiliac preparations (Hubbard et al., 2015). A woman must decide individually whether she can accept these as it is not specifically forbidden to take in tissue or bone from another human. Jehovah's Witnesses currently accept organ transplants, although any surgery would have to be performed on a bloodless basis (Kitahara et al., 2019). The midwife should be aware of the importance of seeking the woman's views on the use of blood products during pregnancy and childbirth. It is crucial to gain to what degree the woman may refuse blood products and prepare the woman for the chances of this eventuality.

JUDAISM AND HEALTH BELIEFS

Judaism holds human life as sacred, having been created by God, who created the matter from which life is made (Eisenberg, 2017). Teachings include caring for one's health and safety, as God can better be served when healthy (Greenberger, 2017). There are no restrictions to required medical treatment in Jewish law due to the guiding principle that the saving of a life is paramount. Therefore, blood transitions and the use of non-Kosher products, such as insulin, is not prohibited. If an individual has a condition that is life-threatening, treatment can be provided without advice from a Rabbi. There are some exceptions to this rule, such as if any treatment results in the death of another person.

ISLAM AND HEALTH BELIEFS

Muslims view health as one of God's greatest blessings bestowed on humankind (Mataoui & Sheldon, 2016). Health has spiritual, physical, emotional and psychological dimensions that involve the well-being of the body, mind and soul (Wehbe-Alamah et al., 2020). Muslims are accountable to God for their health (Rassool, 2014). One's body belongs to God, and therefore, Muslims must care for their bodies (Andrews, 2013). Substances and practices that are harmful to health are forbidden according to Islamic teachings (such as alcohol, illicit drugs, pork products) and engaging in health-promoting practices is encouraged by Islam (such as prayers, meditation, cleanliness, physical fitness, fasting, ablution and breastfeeding) (Wehbe-Alamah et al., 2020). Illness has many interpretations in Islam, such as being a test from God, a natural occurrence, and punishment of sin (Rassool, 2014). Islamic rituals are also followed in pregnancy regarding food and alcohol (Arousell and Carltom, 2016).

HINDUISM AND HEALTH BELIEFS

Hindus believe that all illnesses, whether physical or mental, have a biological, psychological and spiritual element (Sharma, 2002). Treatments that do not address all three causes may not be considered effective by a Hindu patient. Many Hindus attach a stigma to mental illness (Dein et al., 2020) and have a strong belief in the concept of the evil eye and may believe this to be a cause of mental illness. In addition, all illnesses, including mental illness, may be seen as the result of karma from this or a previous life.

Hinduism encourages the acceptance of pain and suffering as part of the consequences of karma. It is not seen as a punishment but as a natural consequence of past negative behaviour and is often seen as an opportunity to progress spiritually. Hindus believe that the time of death is determined by one's destiny and accept death and illness as part of life.

BUDDHISM AND HEALTH BELIEFS

The Buddhist worldview of health and disease states that the overall state of a human being and are interwoven with several non-medical elements, such as economics, education, social and cultural milieu and ethics or morality (Kalra et al., 2018). Health in Buddhism is understood to be achieved by the wholeness of the person involving a holistic approach. Buddhism believes health is achieved with harmony within oneself, in one's social relationships, and in relation to the natural environment (Ratanakul, 2004). To be concerned about a person's health means to be concerned with the whole person: his or her physical, mental and moral dimensions; social, familial and work relationships; as well as the environment in which the person lives (Kalra et al., 2018).

Exercise

A midwife is booking a woman who is having her first baby. During their discussion the woman states she is a Jehovah's Witness.
1. What key information should the midwife discuss with the woman?
2. What key information should the midwife seek from the woman?

Status of the Foetus in Different Religions

THE FOETUS IN CHRISTIANITY

Some religions embrace the belief that an early embryo in vitro constitutes a person, but this belief is not a universal ethical principle. In general, the Roman Catholic Church is the strongest proponent of this belief, and has in recent decades objected to the artificial creation and use of human embryos and human embryonic stem cells in every form (Neaves, 2017). The Catechism of the Catholic Church (1997) states that 'Human life' must be respected and protected from the moment of conception; abortion willed either as an end or means is gravely contrary to the moral law. This is similar to the Church of England, which combines strong opposition to abortion with the recognition that there can be limited conditions under which it may be morally preferable to other alternatives (Church of England, 2021). However, abortion is acceptable by other Christian denominations in the circumstances of rare incest and if there is potential impact on the health of the mother.

THE FOETUS IN ISLAM

Islam respects an embryo because of its potential to grow into a human being but does not assert that a blastocyst is already a person; therefore, there is a distinction between actual life and potential life (Neaves, 2017). Islam has no central authority that determines the status of human embryos, and the pivotal question revolves around the timing of when the foetus is endowed with a soul and the beginning of personhood (Opoku and Manu, 2015). The Koran does not provide an answer, and the Muslim World League has embraced a time point of 120 days after conception (Sivaraman and Noor, 2014). The three stages of development of the foetus are first the semen, second, the blood clot and third, a lump of flesh which are each assigned a 40-day duration. Then it is believed in Islam that an angel is sent, and he breathes the soul into it (Brown, 2004). Following this reasoning, the belief is that aborting the foetus within the first 120 days would be permitted, and Muslims hold the belief that aborting the foetus will be permitted within the first 40 days.

THE FOETUS IN JUDAISM

In Judaism, the embryo is considered to be 'mere water' until the 40th day when a soul may take up residence in the developing body (Ron-El and Rizk, 2012), but there are also beliefs in the Jewish faith that full personhood to a foetus only occurs at birth and assigned as the head is born (Schenker, 2008). In Jewish law, a woman who has had a miscarriage that occurred 40 days after conception is treated as if she has given birth. At any stage in pregnancy, if the mother's life is threatened, and the only way to save her life is a termination of pregnancy, this is permitted and obligatory in Jewish law.

THE FOETUS IN HINDUISM

In Hinduism, the soul is already joined with the matter in the act of conception. The embryo is not just an extension of the mother's flesh but is considered to be an independent soul (Yadav, 2018). It is believed that not being permitted to be born and given the opportunity to do good 'karma', the foetus is done a grave injustice, abortion therefore, violates not only 'karma', but also dharma (virtue) as it forces an 'untimely death' of the foetus (Koley, 2018). The mother is considered to be just a vessel, so the embryo/foetus then is not a private concern of the mother alone, and an abortion is not allowed on that ground (Koley, 2018).

THE FOETUS IN BUDDHISM

Under Buddhist teachings (Buchitchon, 2012), an embryo acquires personhood after implantation in a mother's uterus, at which point consciousness enters the womb. Therefore, termination of pregnancy would be seen as an act of killing, going against Buddhist precepts. Most Buddhists believe in reincarnation, and this belief has a direct impact on Buddhists' views on abortion (Buchitchon, 2012). However, research may be conducted on human embryos in vitro if the intent is to help humankind.

Religion and Spiritual Beliefs Related to Pregnancy and Contraception

AFRICAN RELIGIOUS BELIEFS AND PREGNANCY

Religious and spiritual beliefs strongly influence behaviour over the perinatal period. Religion and health are interrelated, especially within the African context, where illnesses have been linked to spiritual effects (Badoe et al., 2009). In Africa, there is importance of traditional practitioners, such as spiritual healers and religious leaders, as protectors of the pregnancy (Syed et al., 2008; Rees and Yoneda, 2013). During pregnancy, African women intensify their prayers to God for protection, safe delivery and blessings (Jesse et al., 2007). Due to fear of surgery or death during pregnancy, some women explore traditional and spiritual options to ensure a spontaneous vaginal delivery (Aziato et al., 2016). There may be the use of religious artefacts and holy water and oil during pregnancy for protection. Traditional beliefs and practices include food and water restrictions, avoiding burial grounds, avoiding individuals who are deemed to be evil and not going out at specific times of the day.

Christianity and Pregnancy

Generally, pregnancy is received with thanks and praise, under whatever circumstances, a child is believed to be born without sin and is accepted by God. The Catholic Church officially believes that birth control is a violation of natural law and that sexual intercourse is for the express purpose of procreation; any form of contraceptive use is against their religion.

Islam and Pregnancy

In Islam, it is believed that the thoughts and actions of the mother have an impact on the actions and faith of the unborn child. This is because the child is said to be an organ of the mother and obtains all the necessary factors of development from her. Therefore, the prosperity and adversity of a child are determined in the mother's stomach. The pregnancy should only be revealed to close relatives and those who wish good for the mother. This is to ward off the evil eye and envy (hasad). Islam's official stance on birth control is that all forms of it are permissible if both parties consent to its use. However, in reality, the man is the decision-maker in this aspect. Women who identified as Sunni Muslim are less likely to use all forms of contraception than Shia Muslims. Shia Muslim women are more likely to use the birth control pill than other types of contraceptives. However, the Muslim viewpoint on contraception varies, with some followers stating it is prohibited, whereas the main opinion allows contraception, such as oral and injectable contraceptives and condoms (Faraz, 2021).

Judaism and Pregnancy

In Judaism, women are expected to keep the pregnancy a secret during the first trimester in fear of the ayin ha'ra (evil eye). In Jewish law, every woman in the process of childbirth is deemed to be in a life-threatening situation, even for a normal pregnancy. Therefore, any measures that are necessary for childbirth can occur even on the Sabbath or Festivals. In the Jewish faith, childbirth is defined as commencing when the woman can no longer walk unaided or at the commencement of bleeding or regular contractions. Once the process of childbirth has commenced, the obligation to fast on Yom Kippur and other fast days is suspended for 7 days (Webhe-Alamah, 2020).

Most rabbinic authorities believe and teach their followers that women may use contraception, but only certain forms of it. In Judaism, contraceptive methods must enable sexual intercourse to occur and happen without a barrier naturally. So, the pill and other forms of hormonal birth control are generally permitted. Hormonal contraceptive methods are the most acceptable, followed by diaphragms. Male condoms are not allowed. Methods that cause irregular bleeding may be unacceptable because of the requirement for 7 days' sexual abstinence following uterine bleeding. Reversible methods of contraception are preferred as opposed to male and female sterilisation (Weisberg and Kern, 2009).

Buddhism and Pregnancy

In Buddhism, it is believed that the environment of the womb is controlled by the choices the mother makes, which in turn influences the consciousness of the embryo (Damian, 2010). In the Buddhist culture, pregnancy and childbirth are very spiritual processes, and it is believed that a woman who gives birth can walk between two worlds; giving birth is a rite of passage. The woman is expected to surrender to the birth energy but find the connection of the physical, spiritual, and energetic power within herself. The baby inside the womb is a spirit that is taking on flesh. The foetus is believed to dream and think about past lives and considers plans for this new incarnation. This is why the pregnant woman can meditate between the two worlds. The womb symbolises the field of emptiness, which is where all things rise and fall. Buddhists generally object to contraceptive methods that prevent implantation, including intrauterine devices and the emergency contraceptive pill (Harvey, 2000).

Hinduism and Pregnancy

In general, most Hindus believe that the beginning of personhood coincides with the occurrence of reincarnation at the moment of conception and that the earliest human embryo deserves respect (Sivaraman and Noor, 2014). In Hindu, Punsavana—the 'male thinking' rite is performed during the third month of pregnancy, in the belief that the 'deity' governing the sex of the foetus is activated and a male baby will be born. Simmanantannaya, also known as Valaiakappu in some parts of India, involves the wearing of red or green glass bangles from the seventh month of gestation. The sound of these bangles is believed to reach the womb and comfort the foetus. (Gatrad et al., 2004). Hinduism does not take a rigid opinion against contraception (Sharma, 2002).

Practice Point

Exploring the difference between cultural beliefs and values highlights how these interplay with each other. People from the same culture may not have the same beliefs or values, and several factors may affect this. There is also an impact of religion on culture and vice versa, and often the origin of beliefs and values may be a mixture of both components. The next section provides an overview of health beliefs and practices in different cultures.

Bereavement in Different Religions

Several similarities and differences occur in the way Jewish, Christian and Muslim individuals and families observe rituals and care for the dying and dead (Webhe-Alamah et al., 2020). Islamic beliefs and traditions, like those of Christianity and Judaism, define a conceptual framework for an encounter with loss and the ensuing grief. In Table 3.4, rituals relevant to death and bereavement in the event of a late miscarriage, stillbirth or neonatal death are provided.

TABLE 3.4 ■ Death Rituals in Various Religions

Faith	Ritual
Judaism	Shiva, a period of mourning for seven days, 30 days and then annually, is observed. This is not observed for a neonate/infant who has died within 30 days of birth. Autopsies are generally prohibited
Christianity	Practice varies widely between different Christian denominations and around the world. Roman Catholicism and the Orthodox Churches still strongly favour burial over cremation due to a belief in the physical resurrection of the body
Islam	• All children are considered to be innocent. Upon death, the soul of the child will ascend directly to Paradise. This teaching also applies to the baby who has not taken a breath following birth • Miscarried and stillborn babies may be given a name and should be bathed and shrouded • Burial should occur within 24 hours of the time of death
Hinduism	In Hindu at death, the baby is believed to leave the 'earthly' realm into an 'intermediate' zone in readiness for its journey to the 'Divine realm'. Most Hindus are cremated
Buddhism	• There are no universally agreed death or funeral rites prescribed in Buddhism, and Buddhists often follow the common tradition in the country they are living in • Particularly for British converts to Buddhism (rather than British Buddhists from immigrant families), funerals are most likely to take the form of cremation at the local crematorium

Modified from Gatrad, Nemati A., 2005. Abortion from the perspective of law and jurisprudence. *J. Fertil. Reprod.* 4, 369–374. Uzell, J., 2018. Death and funeral rituals in world religions. Available at: https://religionmediacentre.org.uk/factsheets/death-funeral-rituals-in-world-religions/.

Impact of Culture on Health

SYSTEMS OF HEALTH BELIEF

Many cultures have systems of health beliefs to explain the causes of ill health, treatment and prevention. Different cultural groups have diverse belief systems with regard to health and healing in comparison to the Western biomedical model of medicine (Vaughn et al., 2009). These belief systems may include different disease models, wellness/illness paradigms (e.g., Chinese medicine, magico-religious thinking), various culturally specific diseases and disorders, feelings about healthcare providers and seeking Westernised healthcare and the use of traditional and indigenous healthcare practices and approaches (Vaughn et al., 2009). Even in Western cultures, these health beliefs are present. However, Western beliefs attribute ill health to natural scientific phenomena treated with medical technology, which is evidence-based, whereas, in other cultures, ill health may be attributed to supernatural phenomena which can be treated by prayer or spiritual intervention. Health beliefs vary between cultures and individuals within those cultures. Helman (2001) suggests that people attribute causes of illness to:

(1) factors within individuals themselves (e.g., bad habits or negative emotional states)
(2) factors within the natural environment (e.g., pollution and germs)
(3) factors associated with others or the social world (e.g., interpersonal stress, medical facilities and actions of others)
(4) supernatural factors including God, destiny and indigenous beliefs such as witchcraft or voodoo

Awareness and understanding of differences in health beliefs and values between the midwife and the woman are necessary to achieve desired health goals. When caring for women from cultures unfamiliar to the midwife, these differences may need more exploration (Public Health England, 2017). Once the midwife can discuss the expressed beliefs of the woman on differences in response to illness and disease and what influences her health-seeking behaviour and interpretation, this can lead to timely diagnosis. The midwife should always be aware that women's cultural perspectives can be influenced by a range of factors, including ethnicity and place of origin, education, religion, values, gender, age, family and social status.

PARADIGMS OF DISEASE THEORY

The three commonly held paradigms of disease across cultures are naturalistic, personalistic and emotionalistic (Kottak, 2011) (see Table 3.5). Naturalistic theories of illness are more commonly seen in Western cultures and medical practice. Scientific evidence is used to determine the causes of disease, and evidence-based practice is used to treat diseases. In non-Western cultures, personalistic and emotional theories are usually attributed to the cause of illness.

A woman's acceptance of medical advice, including medication use, may be influenced by subjective beliefs about their health condition (Shahin et al., 2019). In some cases, a woman may adhere to two or more theories of ill health and may choose to follow both practices regarding seeking health. For example, a woman may believe in the naturalistic causes of ill health but may have an underlying belief that emotionalistic causes are also relevant. Often family can influence a woman in believing the cause of ill health. When this occurs, the woman may seek health advice from various sources. Therefore it is essential for the midwife to take the women's health beliefs into account when giving health advice on her pregnancy (Hsiao et al., 2012).

TABLE 3.5 ■ Paradigms of Disease Theory

Paradigm	Theory	Principle
Naturalistic (Vaughn et al., 2009)	Naturalistic disease theories explain disease in objective, scientific terms and have the core concept that illness occurs when the body is out of balance	Disease as originating inside the body due to a specific, identifiable 'medical' cause or pathogen (viral, bacterial, etc.)
Personalistic (Helman, 2001)	Geek/Roman origin- healing occurs by restoring the proper balance of humours through removal (bleeding, starvation) or replacing (special diets, medicine) the deficiency	The body contains four elements (humours): blood, phlegm, yellow bile and black bile and health comes from an equal balance of these elements
Emotionalistic (Foster and Anderson, 1978)	Illness is caused by strong emotional states (e.g., intense anger, jealousy, shame, grief or fright). The personalistic and emotionalistic disease theories	Attributes illness to intervention by an agent such as another human, witch, sorcerer, non-human, or supernatural force

Exercise

Review the following scenarios below to further understand how health behaviour in an individual may be influenced by cultural disease theory.

A woman seeks advice from her GP as she is feeling unwell and wants to have tests and investigations to check the cause of her illness.

A woman drinks hot water and begins to fast as she feels unwell; she believes that her illness is due to an internal imbalance.

A woman resorts to prayer and a period of isolation to ward off external influences which she believes are causing her illness.

Learning Activity

After reading the scenarios, state which paradigm of disease model you think could be applied to each scenario. Why is it important for you to understand these disease models when offering health advice to a woman?

Traditional Medicine

In many cultures, traditional medicine (TM) may be used instead of Western medicine. TM has a long history and is defined as the sum of the knowledge, skill and practices based on the theories, beliefs and experiences indigenous to different cultures, used in the maintenance of health as well as in the prevention, diagnosis, improvement or treatment of physical and mental illness (WHO, 2013). According to WHO, 65% to 80% of the world's healthcare practice involves the use of TM, commonly referred to as complementary and alternative medicine (CAM) (WHO, 2013). You will come in contact with women who use TM or alternative therapies and need to be cognisant of the potential impact on the woman and the foetus. Finlayson and Downe (2013), in a systematic review, found that cultural beliefs regarding the need to protect a pregnancy from supernatural threats were combined with women's preferences for TMs in a variety of low- and middle-income countries. Also, there was a commonly held cultural view of pregnancy as a normal physiological state, as opposed to a perception of pregnancy as a risky situation (Barnes et al., 2018). This view may lead women to not seek Western medical advice and to seek out alternative medicine.

CHINESE TRADITIONAL MEDICINE

One of the best-known philosophies that influences ancient East Asian medicine, such as traditional Chinese medicine, is the belief in the opposing forces in the form of *yin and yang* (Dennis et al., 2007; Kim-Godwin, 2003). *Yin* describes properties such as darkness, cold, wetness, softness, quiescence and femininity, while *yang* describes the opposite and includes properties such as brightness, heat, dryness, hardness, activity and masculinity (Dennis et al., 2007). In Chinese TM, yin and yang are considered two types of energy that maintain a homeostatic status in the human body and in the universe; if the homeostasis of yin and yang is broken, the human body will become weak or ill (Liang et al., 2015). Chinese TM also believes in the Five Phase theory, a phase called 'Wu' which refers to the composition of the human body, and the other four phases are the whole universe, which is made of wood, fire, earth, metal and water, and 'XING' refers to special relationships of the 'Wu' elements, which are in constant motion and change (Liang et al., 2015). It is believed that human organs respond to different elements;

for example, the liver, stomach, spleen, lung and kidney respond to wood, fire, earth, metal and water, respectively (Ma et al., 2014; Liang et al., 2015). Practices used in Chinese medicine are acupuncture—use of fine needles gently packed in the skin; cupping—heated cups that create suction on the skin; Herbs—such as teas, powders and capsules mostly made from plants; Moxibustion—dried herbs burned near the skin and mediation. Similarities from traditional Chinese medicine influence many of the dietary practices in Asia, as well as in many other non-Western cultures, including parts of Latin America and Africa (Kim-Godwin, 2003; Dennis et al., 2007).

ANCIENT INDIAN MEDICINE (AYURVEDA)

The ancient Indian medical system, also known as Ayurveda, is based on ancient writings that rely on a 'natural' and holistic approach to physical and mental health (National Center for Complementary and Integrative Health, 2020). Ayurvedic medicine is one of the world's oldest medical systems and remains one of India's traditional healthcare systems. According to Ayurvedic theory, good health requires that there is a balance of three humours: bile (fire), phlegm (water) and wind. Disturbance of this homeostatic condition causes illness, and foods can aggravate a particular humour, causing a loss of balance (Panda, 2017). Blood may be perceived as the life force and treated as precious. Ayurvedic treatment combines products (mainly derived from plants, but may also include animal, metal and mineral), diet, exercise and lifestyle. Several studies also document the widespread use of TMs and herbs among pregnant women in Asian cultures (Withers et al., 2018). Medicines or herbs may be taken orally, used in medicinal baths, enemas, or as ointments; most are commonly used to combat nausea during pregnancy or to stimulate labour (de Boer and Cotingting, 2014; Raman et al., 2014).

AFRICAN TRADITIONAL MEDICINE

Across Africa, herbal remedies are also prevalent, and diagnosis is usually reached through spiritual means before a treatment is prescribed. African traditional healing practices rely on beliefs that existed long before the spread of modern medicine; these practices vary in different African countries (Kubukeli, 1999). Traditional African medicine believes that illness is caused by spiritual or social imbalances. A large number of Africans rely on TMs and believe in spiritual treatments and divination (Mattelaer, 2005). These beliefs are maintained despite colonisation, and what occurs is a mix of Western medicine and African TM practices, which persist despite acculturation. Optimum health for Africans constitutes mental, physical, spiritual and emotional stability for oneself and their families (Omonzejele, 2008). This may lead to a woman seeking cures for various symptoms in pregnancy from multiple sources.

ARABIAN MEDICINE

The use of Arabic medicine is also prevalent in the Middle East and Southeast Asia. In traditional Arabic medicine, a large variety of plants is used for the treatment of various diseases in the form of herbal teas, syrups, infusions and ointments (Saad et al., 2005). A commonly used herb, *Nigella sativa* (L.), also known as black seed, is used both as an herb and oil for the prevention and cure of many ailments (Al-Ghamdi, 2001), including respiratory health, immune system support and stomach and intestinal health (Gupta et al., 2009). The use of honey is also common in Arabic medicine. Honey's medicinal use encompasses a wide range of concerns, including promoting circulation, eliminating stomach and intestinal pain and colic and as a topical antibiotic (Oumeish, 1998).

Practice Point

A discussion of any medicine a woman may be taking during pregnancy also needs to include any traditional medicine. An exploration with the woman of potential harm from any traditional medicine can lead to the woman understanding why some medicines should be avoided. Adopting this culturally aware and sensitive approach prevents the woman from not divulging information that you can use to provide informed choices.

REFLECTIVE QUESTIONS

1. Why is it important to have knowledge about a woman's cultural beliefs?
2. Think about how religious beliefs can impact a woman's choices in pregnancy.
3. What role does the woman's belief of causes of ill health play in pregnancy health?
4. What factors would you need to consider if a woman was using tradition medicines in pregnancy?

References

Abdulla, M.R., 2018. Culture, religion, and freedom of religion or belief. Rev. Faith Int. Aff. 16 (4), 102–115.

Alexiou, E., 2016. Fasting, the orthodox Christian way. Orthodox Christian Network., Available at. http://myocn.net/fasting-the-orthodox-christian-way/.

Al-Ghamdi, M.S., 2001. The anti-inflammatory, analgesic and antipyretic activity of Nigella sativa. J. Ethnopharmacol. 76 (1), 45–48.

Andrews, J., 2013. Cultural, ethnic, and religious references manual for healthcare providers, 4th ed. JAMARDA Resources, Winston-Salem, NC.

Arthington, M., 2019. The difference between Shiite and Sunni Muslims and why it matters. International Mission Board. Available at. https://www.imb.org/2019/05/24/difference-between-shiite-sunni-muslims/.

Arousell, J., Carlbom, A., 2016. Culture and religious beliefs in relation to reproductive health. Best Pract. Res. Clin. Obstet. Gynaecol 32, 77–87.

Aziato, L., Odai, P.N., Omenyo, C.N., 2016. Religious beliefs and practices in pregnancy and labour: an inductive qualitative study among post-partum women in Ghana. BMC Pregnancy and Childbirth 16 (1), 1–10.

Badoe, E.A., Archampong, E.Q., da Rocha-Afodu, J.T., 2009. A brief history of surgery. Principles and practice of surgery including pathology in the tropics. Tema: Ghana Publishing Corp. 1–11.

Barnes, L.A.J., Barclay, L., McCaffery, K., Aslani, P., 2018. Complementary medicine products used in pregnancy and lactation and an examination of the information sources accessed pertaining to maternal health literacy: a systematic review of qualitative studies. BMC Complement. Altern. Med. 18 (1), 229.

Beckford, J.A., Demerath, J. (Eds.), 2007. The SAGE Handbook of the Sociology of Religion Sage, London.

Bell, C., 1997. Ritual: Perspectives and Dimensions. Oxford University Press, New York. p. 94.

Beyers, J., 2017. Religion and culture: Revisiting a close relative. HTS Teol. Stud. 73 (1), 1–9.

Brown, D.E., 2004. Human universals, human nature & human culture. Daedalus 133 (4), 47–54.

Buchitchon, S., 2012. Buddhism and the status of the human embryo: the regulation of human embryo research in Thailand. La Trobe University, Victoria.

Catechism of the Catholic Church, 1997. Revised in Accordance with the Official Latin Text Promulgated by Pope John Paul II, second ed. Libreria Editrice Vaticana, Vatican City.

Chae, C., Okocha, O., Sweitzer, B., 2020. Preoperative considerations for Jehovah's witness patients: a clinical guide. Curr Opin Anaesthesiol. 33 (3), 432–440.

Church of England. 2021. Abortion statement. Available at: https://www.churchofengland.org/sites/default/files/2017-11/Abortion%20Church%20of%20England%20Statements.pdf (accessed January 2021).

Cohen, A.B., Varnum, M.E., 2016. Beyond east vs. west: social class, region, and religion as forms of culture. Curr. Opin. Psychol. 8, 5–9.

Crowther, S., Hall, J., 2015. Spirituality and spiritual care in and around childbirth. Women Birth 28 (2), 173–178.

Damian, C.I., 2010. Abortion from the perspective of eastern religions: Hinduism and Buddhism. Revista Romana de Bioetica 8 (1), 124–136.

Darkwah, A.K., 2016. Globalisation, development and the empowerment of women: the case of African traders. In: Handbook on gender in world politics. Edward Elgar Publishing, Cheltenham, UK.

De Boer, H.J., Cotingting, C., 2014. Medicinal plants for women's healthcare in southeast Asia: a meta-analysis of their traditional use, chemical constituents, and pharmacology. J. Ethnopharmacol. 151 (2), 747–767.

Dein, S., Persaud, A., Tribe, R., Bhugra, D., Bhui, K., Lashley, M., et al., 2020. Moving beyond Christianity: Islam, Judaism, Hinduism and mental health. World Cult. Psychiatry Res. Rev. 14 (1–2), 13–19.

Dennis, C.L., Fung, K., Grigoriadis, S., Robinson, G.E., Romans, S., Ross, L., 2007. Traditional postpartum practices and rituals: a qualitative systematic review. Women's Health 3 (4), 487–502.

Department of Health (DOH), 2009. Religion or belief: a practical guide for the NHS. The national archives. Available at: https://webarchive.nationalarchives.gov.uk/ukgwa/20130123195548/http://www.dh.gov.uk/en/Publicationsandstatistics/Publications/PublicationsPolicyAndGuidance/DH_093133.

Eisenberg, D., 2017. Maintaining compassion for the suffering terminal patient while preserving life: an orthodox Jewish approach. Perspect. Biol. Med. 60 (2), 233–246.

Emmanuel, S.M., 2013. A Companion to Buddhist Philosophy: Blackwell Companions to Philosophy. John Wiley & Sons, Oxford.

Erwin, R.G., Haemig, M.J., Jones, K.S., Lohrmann, M.J., Nelson, D.R., Stjerna, K.I., Wengert, T.J., Wiersma, H., 2017. By heart: Conversations with Martin Luther's Small Catechism. Augsburg Fortress., Available at: https://www.augsburgfortress.org/store/product/9781506431482/By-Heart-Conversations-with-Martin-Luthers-Small-Catechism.

Faraz, A., 2012. Is contraception permissible in Islam? Darul Fiqh Available at: https://darulfiqh.com/is-contraception-permissible-in-islam-2/.

Finlayson, K., Downe, S., 2013. Why do women not use antenatal services in low-and middle-income countries? A meta-synthesis of qualitative studies. PLoS Med. 10 (1), e1001373.

Foster, G.M., Anderson, B.G., 1978. Medical Anthropology. McGraw Hill, New York.

Gatrad, A.R., Ray, M., Sheikh, A., 2004. Hindu birth customs. Arch Dis Child. 89 (12), 1094–1097.

Gaygısız, Ü., Lajunen, T., Gaygısız, E., 2017. Socio-economic factors, cultural values, national personality and antibiotics use: a cross-cultural study among European countries. Journal of infection and public health. 10 (6), 7553–7760.

Goddard, N.C., 1995. Spirituality as integrative energ': a philosophical analysis as requisite precursor to holistic nursing practice. J. Adv. Nurs. 22 (4), 808–815.

Goodwin, R., Marshall, T., Fülöp, M., Adonu, J., Spiewak, S., Neto, F., et al., 2012. Mate value and self-esteem: Evidence from eight cultural groups. PLoS One 7 (4), e36106.

Green, A., 1997. Folklore: An Encyclopedia of Beliefs, Customs, Tales, Music, and Art. ABC-CLIO, Santa Barbara, CA, ISBN 978-0-87436-986-1.

Greenberger, C., 2017. Religion, Judaism, and the challenge of maintaining an adequately immunized population. Nurs. Ethics 24 (6), 653–662.

Greer, D.B., Abel, W.M., 2017. Religious/spiritual coping in older African American women. Qual. Rep. 22 (1), 237.

Gupta, S., Jhade, D., Ahirwar, D., Sharma, N.K., 2009. Medicinal and pharmacological potentials of Nigella sativa. Ethnobotanical Rev. 946–955.

Harvey, P., 2000. An Introduction to Buddhist Ethics: Foundations, Values and Issues. Cambridge University Press, Cambridge.

Harvey, P., 2013. An Introduction to Buddhism: Teachings, History and Practices, second ed. Cambridge University Press, Cambridge.

Hatah, E., Lim, K.P., Ali, A.M., Shah, N.M., Islahudin, F., 2015. The influence of cultural and religious orientations on social support and its potential impact on medication adherence. Patient Prefer. Adherence 9, 589.

Helman, C.G., 2001. Culture, Health and Illness. Arnold, London.

Hofstede, G., 1991. Empirical models of cultural differences. In: Bleichrodt, N., Drenth, P.J.D. (Eds.), Contemporary issues in cross-cultural psychology. Swets & Zeitlinger Publishers, pp. 4–20.

Hofstede, G., 2010. Culture's consequences: comparing values, behaviors, institutions, and organizations across nations, second ed. Sage Publications, Thousand Oaks, CA.

Hofstede, G., 2011. Dimensionalizing cultures: The Hofstede model in context. ORPC. 2 (1) 2307-0919.

Hofstede, G., Hofstede, G.J., Minkov, M., 2010. Cultures and organizations: software of the mind, vol. 3. McGraw-Hill, New York.

Hordern, J., 2016. Religion, culture and conscience. Medicine. 44 (10), 589–592. Available at: https://www.sciencedirect.com/science/article/pii/S1357303916301438.

Hsiao, C.Y., Chang, C., Chen, C.D., 2012. An investigation on illness perception and adherence among hypertensive patients. Kaohsiung J Med Sci. 28 (8), 442–447.

Hubbard, R., Waters, J.H., Yazer, M.H., 2015. Heterogeneity in blood product acceptance among antenatal patients of the Jehovah's witness faith. Obstet. Gynecol. 126 (5), 974–977.

Idang, G.E., 2015. African culture and values. Phronimon 16 (2), 97–111.

Jesse, D.E., Schoneboom, C., Blanchard, A., 2007. The effect of faith or spirituality in pregnancy: A content analysis. J. Holist. Nurs. 25 (3), 151–158.

Kalra, S., Priya, G., Grewal, E., Aye, T.T., Waraich, B.K., SweLatt, T., et al., 2018. Lessons for the Health-care Practitioner from Buddhism. Indian J. Endocrinol. Metab. 22 (6), 812–817. https://doi.org/10.4103/ijem.IJEM_286_17.

Kim-Godwin, Y.S., 2003. Postpartum beliefs and practices among non-Western cultures. MCN Am. J. Matern. Child Nurs. 28 (2), 74–78.

Kitahara, H., Ota, T., Jeevanandam, V., 2019. Complex Cardiac Surgery Without Blood Transfusions: Lessons Learned from Managing Jehovah Witness Patients. In: Difficult Decisions in Cardiothoracic Critical Care Surgery. Springer, Cham, pp. 499–508.

Koley, K., 2018. Hindus and abortion: A traditional view. Int. J. Creat. Res. Thoughts 6 (2), 92–98.

Kottak, C.P., 2011. Cultural anthropology: appreciating cultural diversity. McGraw-Hill, New York, NY.

Kubukeli, P.S., 1999. Traditional healing practice using medicinal herbs. Lancet, 354. SIV24.

Lepherd, L., 2015. Spirituality: Everyone has it, but what is it? Int. J. Nurs. Pract. 21 (5), 566–574.

Lewinson, L.P., McSherry, W., Kevern, P., 2015. Spirituality in pre-registration nurse education and practice: A review of the literature. Nurse Educ. Today 35 (6), 806–814.

Liang, B., Li, L., Tang, L.Y., Wu, Q., Wu, X.K., Wang, C.C., 2015. Safety of Chinese herbal medicines during pregnancy. J. Appl. Toxicol. 35 (5), 447–458.

Lipner, J., 2004. On Hinduism and Hinduisms: The Way of the Banyan. The Hindu World. Routledge, London, pp. 21–46.

Ma, Z., Jia, C., Guo, J., Gu, H., Miao, Y., 2014. Features analysis of five-element theory and its basal effects on construction of visceral manifestation theory. J. Tradit. Chin. Med. 34 (1), 115–121.

MacKay, D.B., 2000. Ethnicity. In: Braun, W., McCutcheon, R.T. (Eds.), Guide to the Study of Religion. Cassell, London, pp. 96–109.

Marsh, J.C., Bevan, D.H., 2002. Haematological care of the Jehovah's Witness patient. Br. J. Haematol. 119 (1), 25–37.

Mataoui, F.Z., Sheldon, L.K., 2016. Providing culturally appropriate care to American Muslims with cancer. Clin. J. Oncol. Nurs. 20 (1), 11–12.

Mattelaer, J.J., 2005. The aging male in African ethnic cultures. Aging Male 8 (1), 42–47.

National Center for Complementary and Integrative Health, 2020. Ayurvedic Medicine Depth https://www.nccih.nih.gov/health/ayurvedic-medicine-in-depth.

Neaves, W., 2017. The status of the human embryo in various religions. Development 144 (14), 2541–2543.

Omonzejele, P.F., 2008. African concepts of health, disease, and treatment: an ethical inquiry. Explore 4 (2), 120–126.

Opoku, J.K., Manu, E., 2015. The status of the human embryo: an analysis from the Christian and Islamic viewpoints. Eur. J. Biol. Med. Sci. Res. 3 (3), 24–60.

Oumeish, O.Y., 1998. The philosophical, cultural, and historical aspects of complementary, alternative, unconventional, and integrative medicine in the Old World. Arch. Dermatol. 134 (11), 1373–1386.

Panda, D., 2017. Health and Disease in Ayurveda. From Ayurveda to Chinese Medicine, 77–93.

Plante, T.G., Sherman, A.C., (Eds.), 2001. Faith and health: psychological perspectives. Guilford Press.

Popovsky, R.M.A., 2010. Special issues in the care of ultra-orthodox Jewish psychiatric in-patients. Transcult. Psychiatry 47 (4), 647–672.

Public Health England. 2017. Migrant Health Guide. Available at: https://www.gov.uk/topic/health-protection/migrant-health-guide.

Purnell, L.D., 2014. Guide to culturally competent health care. FA Davis, Philadelphia.

Ramadan, T., 2010. What I Believe. Oxford University Press, Oxford.

Raman, S., Srinivasan, K., Kurpad, A., Razee, H., Ritchie, J., 2014. 'Nothing special, everything is Maamuli': socio-cultural and family practices influencing the perinatal period in urban India. PLoS One 9 (11), e111900.

Rassool, G.H. (Ed.), 2014. Cultural Competence in Caring for Muslim Patients. Macmillan International Higher Education, New York.

Ratanakul, P., 2004. Buddhism, health and disease. Eubios J. Asian Int. Bioeth. 15, 162–164.

Rees, G., Yoneda, F., 2013. Celibate monks and foetus-stealing gods: Buddhism and pregnancy at the Jetavana Monastery, Shravasti, India. World Archaeol. 45 (2), 252–271.

Regenstein, J.M., Chaudry, M.M., Regenstein, C.E., 2003. The kosher and halal food laws. Compr. Rev. Food Sci. Food Saf. 2 (3), 111–127.

Ron-El, R., Rizk, B., 2012. Religious perspectives in human reproduction In: Textbook of Assisted Reproductive Techniques, pp. 451–456.

Rush, R.A., Aboul-Enein, B.H., 2016. Health, Healing, and weel-being according to the New Testament. ABNF J. 27 (2), 44–47.

Saad, B., Azaizeh, H., Said, O., 2005. Tradition and perspectives of Arab herbal medicine: a review. Evid. Based Complement. Alternat. Med. 2, 475–479.

Sábaté, R.S., Gelabert, R., Badilla, Y., Del Valle, C., 2016. Feeding holy bodies: A study on the social meanings of a vegetarian diet to Seventh-day Adventist church pioneers. HTS Teol. Stud. 72 (3).

Savitri, A.I., Yadegari, N., Bakker, J., van Ewijk, R.J., Grobbee, D.E., Painter, R.C., et al., 2014. Ramadan fasting and newborn's birth weight in pregnant Muslim women in The Netherlands. Br. J. Nutr. 112 (9), 1503–1509.

Schenker, J.G., 2008. The beginning of human life. J. Assist. Reprod. Genet. 25 (6), 271–276.

Schief, M., Lin, Q., Haenni, S., 2018. Harmful Traditional Practices: Child Marriage, Initiation Rituals, FGM/C. Center for Child Well-Being and Development, pp. 1–76.

Schlegel, A., Barry III, H., 1980. The evolutionary significance of adolescent initiation ceremonies. Am. Ethnol. 7 (4), 696–715.

Schlegel, A., Barry III, H., 2017. Pain, fear, and circumcision in boys' adolescent initiation ceremonies. Cross Cult. Res. 51 (5), 435–463.

Schwartz, S.H., 2012. An overview of the Schwartz theory of basic values. ORPC. 2 (1), 2307-0919.

Shahin, W., Kennedy, G.A., Stupans, I., 2019. The impact of personal and cultural beliefs on medication adherence of patients with chronic illnesses: a systematic review. Patient Prefer. Adherence 13, 1019–1035.

Sharma, A., 2000. Classical Hindu Thought. Oxford University Press, Oxford, p. 72.

Sharma, A., 2002. The Hindu tradition: Religious beliefs, and healthcare decisions. Religious Traditions and Healthcare Decisions, The Park Ridge Center for the Study of Health, Faith and Ethics, pp. 1–20.

Shils, E., 1981. Tradition. University of Chicago Press, Chicago.

Sivaraman, M.A.F., Noor, S.N.M., 2014. Ethics of embryonic stem cell research according to Buddhist, Hindu, Catholic, and Islamic religions: perspective from Malaysia. Asian Biomed. 8 (1), 43–52.

Stefon, M., 2020. Christianity. Available at: https://www.britannica.com/topic/Christianity.

Swihart, D.L., Yarrarapu, S.N.S., Martin, R.L., 2021. Cultural religious competence in clinical practice StatPearls [Internet]. StatPearls Publishing, Treasure Island (FL).

Syed, U., Khadka, N., Khan, A., Wall, S., 2008. Care-seeking practices in South Asia: using formative research to design program interventions to save newborn lives. J. Perinatol. 28 (2), S9–S13.

Tieman, M., Hassan, F.H., 2015. Convergence of food systems: Kosher, Christian and Halal. Br. Food J. 117 (9), 2313–2327.

Tyler, S.A., 1973. India: An Anthropological Perspective. Goodyear Publishing Company, California.

Umoh, J.O., 2005. Elements of Sociology of Religion. Iwoh Publishers, Ikot Ekpene.

UNESCO, 2020. Social practices, rituals and festive events. Available at: https://ich.unesco.org/en/social-practices-rituals-and-00055.

Vaughn, L.M., Jacquez, F., Bakar, R.C., 2009. Cultural health attributions, beliefs, and practices: Effects on healthcare and medical education. Open Med. Educ. J. 2 (1), 64–74.

Wehbe-Alamah, H., Hammonds, L.S., Stanley, D., 2020. Culturally congruent care from the perspectives of Judaism, Christianity, and Islam. J. Transcult. Nurs. 32 (2), 119–128.

Weisberg, E., Kern, I., 2009. Judaism and women's health. J. Fam. Plann. Reprod. Health Care 35 (1), 53–55.

Withers, M., Kharazmi, N., Lim, E., 2018. Traditional beliefs and practices in pregnancy, childbirth and post-partum: A review of the evidence from Asian countries. Midwifery 56, 158–170.

World Health Organization, 2013. WHO traditional medicine strategy: 2014-2023. World Health Organization.

Yadav, G., 2018. Abortion (Hinduism). In: Jain, P., Sherma, R., Khanna, M. (Eds.), Hinduism and Tribal Religions. Encyclopedia of Indian Religions. Springer, Dordrecht. https://doi.org/10.1007/978-94-024-1036-5-484-1.

Yen, S., 2020. Birth control and religion. Available at: https://www.pandiahealth.com/resources/birth-control-religion/.

Transcultural Care and Pregnancy

INTRODUCTION

In this chapter the broad values and beliefs of global perspectives of pregnancy and midwifery care within some cultures will be explored. This will inform the reader of the many childbearing practices that women perform and adhere to due to cultural and religious beliefs. The application of culturally competent care and cultural safety in midwifery care provision will be discussed and how this may be affected by personal, professional and organisational culture.

Global Perspectives of Pregnancy and Midwifery Care

In Chapter 1, we discussed the importance of cultural knowledge. Midwives working with women from different cultures will acquire cultural knowledge, particularly if they have regular contact with women. This knowledge can be used to sensitively care for women and it also increases a midwife's cultural awareness. Differences between the cultures of healthcare service providers and service users have been recognised as a major issue in service delivery. Perceived or actual cultural insensitivity or incompetence of professionals can lead to perceptions of poor-quality care by women or discrimination of women by providers, resulting in a lack of trust in services and service providers (Glei et al., 2003; Gabrysch et al., 2009; Esegbona-Adeigbe, 2018).

Midwives can reduce cultural insensitivity by recognising that the woman has her own cultural identity and being aware of how cultural practices around pregnancy are different around the world. It is impossible to acquire cultural knowledge for every culture but what is possible is to understand there are differences and to be able to transgress and discuss these differences when caring for women in any context. Having some insight into different childbirth and pregnancy practices equips the midwife with the first step in closing the gap and creating trust with women. In order to address this issue and promote culturally safe care, it is important to develop knowledge about how women culturally construct their understanding of pregnancy (DeSouza, 2014). This section discusses the broad cultural themes found in different continents and regions globally on pregnancy and how these should be considered in provision of midwifery care.

Pregnancy in Different Cultures

Childbirth is a biological event, however, the social construct surrounding pregnancy is shaped by cultural perceptions and practices (Kaphle et al., 2013; Withers et al., 2018). It is essential as a midwife to understand the relevance of cultural values and beliefs and why they may be adhered to particularly in pregnancy. Beliefs, values and rituals around pregnancy and birth may all impact on a woman's health/health-seeking behaviour, as in traditional societies childbearing is the most important role in a woman's life (Sperstad and Werner, 2005). There are various rituals and practices that exist to protect the mother and unborn child which are practised in numerous cultures around the world. Women who migrate to other countries may adhere to these rituals and practices because of the fear of harm to their pregnancy. The challenges of continuing to obey the practices dictated by culture can be difficult in the diaspora (Esegbona-Adeigbe, 2011). Refugees or newly arrived immigrants may particularly face challenges during pregnancy due to Western influences which may challenge their cultural beliefs whilst adapting to a new environment (Esegbona-Adeigbe, 2011).

The influences of external factors on women's behaviour during pregnancy varies depending on her cultural background. In North America and Western and Eastern Europe factors such as national, state and local laws usually contribute to activities practised during childbirth or a loss after pregnancy (Paul and Iyioriobhe, 2017). However, organisational factors and community relationships play a role in the birth activities practised in parts of Asia and South America, whereas religious factors, interpersonal and individual factors have been identified in Africa (Paul and Iyioriobhe, 2017). Cultural differences are likely to be more persistent than language needs in immigrant groups. According to Szczepura (2005), these might include:

Patient's health, healing and wellness belief systems.

How illness, disease and their causes are perceived.

The behaviour of patients seeking healthcare and their attitudes to healthcare providers.

The views and values of those delivering healthcare.

The beliefs in some cultures surrounding a routine, uncomplicated pregnancy provide a different picture than that commonly shared within Westernised institutional medical practices. Risks or problems during pregnancy may therefore go undiagnosed for longer, the different viewpoint causing delays in women seeking care from maternity services and resorting to more familiar informal sources (Morrison et al., 2014; Withers et al., 2018). Women may also lack knowledge on the importance of maternity care or what attention needs to be paid to pregnancy. This is due to the different set-up of pregnancy care in their own country. Cultural beliefs that conflict with Western beliefs of pregnancy may make it difficult for women to engage with health services. Therefore, knowledge of these cultural beliefs is vital particularly if midwives have frequent contact with women from different cultures. As already discussed there may be cultural practices undertaken that are harmful as they prevent women from seeking health advice or they may indeed be non-detrimental. The lack of knowledge of these practices makes it difficult for midwives to give advice that does not conflict with a woman's cultural beliefs and values (Esegbona-Adeigbe, 2011).

Techno Centric and Ethnokinship Cultures

Posmontier and Horowitz (2007) discusses the two cultural classifications of Western (techno centric) and non-Western (ethnokinship) populations. Techno centric cultures use technology to monitor the new mother and baby. Technological rituals consist of obtaining vital signs, separation of mother and baby and early discharge from the hospital to a social system that does not have any formalised norms or traditions to support the new mother (Dike, 2013). Hence, the woman's status as a new mother is not revered. It is suggested by Posmontier and Horowitz (2007) that a techno centric culture occurs primarily in the United States, Canada, UK, Western Europe and Australia, stating that new mothers are not celebrated in techno centric cultures thus the woman's rite of passage to motherhood is denied.

Ethnokinship culture of childbirth is referred to as one in which the performance of social support rituals by family and communities are the main focus of the postnatal period (Dike, 2013). Ethnokinship culture is said to exist in African, Arabian, Amish, Chinese, Japanese and Mexican cultures (Posmontier and Horowitz, 2007). The mother is supported by being confined and told to rest, given assistance with housework and help with caring for her baby. The mother is revered, honoured and celebrated in ethnokinship cultures and her status is valued. Therefore, in non-Western cultures, the transition to motherhood is supported by family and community who play a significant role. The importance of awareness of these cultural practices by midwives facilitates support for woman and ensures that midwifery care is provided around these cultural norms. In addition, it is essential to be aware of the cultural myths surrounding pregnancy and how perceived risk guides women's behaviour.

Philosophy of Risk in Pregnancy in Different Cultures

Many cultures believe in supernatural influences, either benevolent or malevolent, affecting pregnancy or childbirth. Practices surrounding pregnancy are particularly revered as healthy off springs ensure the survival of family lines. In most traditional societies, while men and women believe equally in malevolent spirits, the belief in harm seems to occur mainly amongst females. Ritual restrictions placed on women through the perinatal period are practised widely across Asia, Africa and parts of Latin America and involve food, sexual intercourse, physical activity and women's mobility (Raman et al., 2014).

The notion of impurities and ritual pollution remains strong in traditional communities, the management of 'impurities' being essential to prevent misfortune in the family (Raman et al., 2016). Superstitious beliefs about pregnancy and childbirth are also found in several Asian countries (Choudhury et al., 2012; Kaphle et al., 2013; Vallely et al., 2013). Purifications and rituals in some Asian cultures are believed to protect a birthing woman from evil spirits complicating childbirth (Vallely et al., 2013). This sort of similar worldview was evident not only in more traditional societies in Asia, but in Africa and Latin America.

Several studies have also documented that in Asia, pregnancy is widely viewed as a natural phenomenon and not as a risky condition (Agus et al., 2012; Syed et al., 2008). The idea of 'pregnancy being 'natural' potentially normalises danger signs in childbirth such as swelling, headaches and small abdominal size (Raman et al., 2016), leading to women not seeking advice when needed. However, women in Asian countries follow traditional practices even though they do not necessarily appreciate their importance, because they are worried about potential negative consequences (to both the baby and mother) if they do not adhere to these customs (Agus et al., 2012; Naser et al., 2012). The fear is that the woman will be blamed if there is a negative outcome to the pregnancy.

Fear of bewitchment is strong in parts of Africa resulting in pregnancy being entirely concealed (Raman et al., 2016). Very little preparation will be made prior to the birth itself as it is believed that performing acts such as naming a child, buying clothes or preparing food is overly optimistic. For this reason pregnancy will not be mentioned until the point at which it becomes noticeable. In Arabian/Middle Eastern cultures pregnancy is never announced shortly after a woman gets pregnant. Women have stated that announcing a pregnancy this early might evoke the evil eye and cause harm to the new mother and her unborn baby (Kridli et al., 2013). As a result, women usually wait until the end of the first trimester to announce the pregnancy, especially if it is the mother's first pregnancy. In Christian, Jewish and Islamic traditions childbirth is regarded as a spiritual experience. It is believed that pregnancy is a time to grow closer to God and the use of religious beliefs and rituals are powerful coping mechanisms (Callister and Khalaf, 2010). Childbirth is also believed to be a time to make religiosity more meaningful and that the significance of a higher power influences birth outcomes (DeVito, 2019).

Practice Point

Awareness of the issues and opposing views regarding risk in pregnancy is important knowledge for midwives; care should be taken to explore these matters with women. These perceived risks in pregnancy can impact women accessing or engaging with pregnancy care. Recommendations that the antenatal booking should be completed as early as 8 weeks can cause conflict with women as they may not wish to reveal their pregnancy at this early stage. Therefore, it is important to stress to women that early booking can help in reducing risk in pregnancy by providing screening, monitoring and early referral to obstetric care if needed. Advice offered by midwives may conflict with women's perception of risk and may have impact on all stages of pregnancy, hence a sensitive discussion of these issues is needed.

Diet During Pregnancy

HOT AND COLD FOOD CONCEPTS DURING PREGNANCY

In many cultures, certain foods are especially encouraged to promote healing or restore health, while other foods are avoided for fear of causing ill health. Food taboos are continued during pregnancy up to the birth of the baby and the postnatal period. Hot/cold beliefs of food are common among traditional cultures in the Middle East, Africa and Asia (Kim-Godwin, 2003; Withers et al., 2018). Physiological changes during pregnancy are believed to cause a hot/cold imbalance in the body, with pregnancy itself considered to be an over-heated state and the postnatal period a cold state. 'Cold' foods are believed to help correct this imbalance during pregnancy and avoid adverse pregnancy outcomes (Callister et al., 2011; Naser et al., 2012), clear toxins and reduce heat. Generally, foods are avoided during pregnancy because of three possible reasons: miscarriage, difficulty in labour and fear of an abnormality in the baby (Chakrabarti and Chakrabarti, 2019).

Cold foods are avoided and hot foods are encouraged during the first month postpartum in Asian cultures (Withers et al., 2018). For example, vegetables and raw fruit are avoided in Chinese women as they are believed to cause an imbalance of 'qi' (lifeforce) leading to sore back muscles, circulatory problems and a weak bladder and uterus. Hot foods are considered to be suitable for the postnatal period to aid healing and involution of the uterus. Examples of hot foods are spicy foods and coffee and milk. Warm or hot foods are believed to raise the body's inner heat, improve the circulation and nourish the energy of the body. Hot and cold food practices can prevent a woman from maintaining a healthy diet during pregnancy which is an important consideration for midwifery care. For example, the concept of 'hot' and 'cold' is widespread in Mexico, where many indigenous women are warned not to eat nutritious foods like tomatoes, eggs and avocados (Adamson, 2015).

In Asian cultures hot and cold food practices are also prevalent. Yoghurt and vegetables, especially gourds (except brinjals and cabbage), are considered to be cold foods and hot foods include papaya, banana, coconut, pineapple, red chilies, jackfruit, meat and egg (Chakrabarti and Chakrabarti, 2019). Cold foods are particularly restricted in the postnatal period due to belief that they could cause a cold in the baby and reduce milk supply in the mother. The hot/cold balance in food and nutrition is also practiced in Caribbean cultures to maintain a healthy physical and mental balance (Volpato and Godinez, 2006).

A study by Xie et al. (2020) confirmed that the cold/hot properties of foods can be linked to their compositions (Fig. 4.1). Energy substances including protein, carbohydrate and lipids significantly contribute to the hot nature of food, as they mainly provide energy to maintain body function as opposed to foods lacking energy substances. So, following the hot/cold food beliefs can have some benefits to the woman.

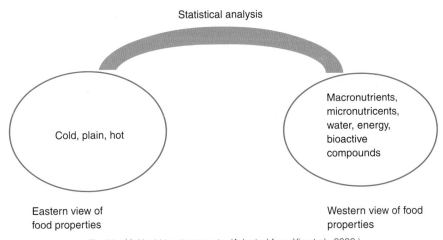

Fig. 4.1 Hot/cold food concepts. (Adapted from Xie et al., 2020.)

FOOD RESTRICTIONS

Food recommendations and restrictions in pregnancy are sometimes based on beliefs regarding the effects they have on the growth of the baby (Mukhopadhyay and Sarkar, 2009; Culhane-Pera et al., 2015). In parts of Asia, Africa and Latin America, food taboos can prevent women from eating a balanced diet and deprive them of essential nutrients (Adamson, 2015). This is again particularly relevant if adhering to food taboos removes elements of a healthy diet such as fruits and vegetables. Common beliefs about certain natural products to be harmful during pregnancy have been observed among pregnant Arabian women although, though there is no established evidence about their risk to pregnancy (Aljoher et al., 2018). For example, the most common reason for food avoidance is fear of its effect on the foetus in Arabian women; cinnamon and pineapple are the most commonly believed products to be harmful during pregnancy (Aljoher et al., 2018). In India, there is a belief that foods should be avoided in the postnatal period. These include certain varieties of green leafy vegetables, fibrous vegetables, melons, pumpkin, papaya, eggplant, shellfish, eggs (in certain castes and communities), certain varieties of fish, lemons, limes, oranges, grapes, chillies, bell peppers, spices, bananas, yoghurt and oily food (Bandyopadhyay, 2009).

Food restrictions are also practised in the Caribbean, with some food cravings believed to mark the child. For example, in Jamaica, if a mother has a craving for mangoes the baby is believed to likely be born with a birthmark resembling a mango.

In China, some symbolic foods are avoided because they are believed to affect the baby's character or appearance (Lau, 2012). For example, eating snacks is believed to be bad for the baby's skin, mutton will cause epilepsy and dark foods are thought to give a baby a darker complexion. In sub-Saharan Africa food restrictions are also followed in pregnancy to avoid a poor pregnancy outcome (Chakona and Shackleton, 2019). For example, in Nigeria, Gambia and Ethiopia pregnant women are usually forbidden from consuming the richest food sources of iron, carbohydrates, animal proteins and micronutrients, mainly because of the fear that the child may develop bad habits after birth or may be born with diseases or the food will cause a delay in labour due to a large baby (Martínez Pérez and Pascual García, 2013; Ugwa, 2016; Vasilevski and Carolan-Olah, 2016).

Practice Point

The midwife should always consider the woman's cultural practices when giving advice on diet. During the booking interview when offering advice on eating a healthy well-balanced diet this should be culturally specific. The simplest method is to begin with asking the woman about her usual daily diet and how food is prepared. If the midwife has some cultural or religious knowledge of dietary practices, e.g., Kosher or Halal, this can assist in advising women of any dietary practices that may impact on pregnancy such as fasting or avoiding foods that contribute to a well-balanced diet.

Medicine Use During Pregnancy

Medicine use in pregnancy is also affected by culture and often traditional medicine is used rather than Western medicine. In some cultures women may fear using any type of medicine during pregnancy due to believed risk to the baby. However, if traditional medicines are used by women during pregnancy these may be harmful.

MEDICINE USE IN PREGNANCY IN AFRICA

Use of traditional medicines for maternity-related health complaints is common in African women (Frawley et al., 2013). Some of the reasons these medicines are used to treat pregnancy-related conditions including nausea, vomiting, swollen feet, back pain, fever, cold, abdominal pain, oedema, urinary tract infection, tiredness and headaches (Shewamene et al., 2017). African traditional medicine is rooted within cultures, with information handed down from close family members (Abdullahi, 2011). The fact that there are several plants used in African traditional medicine, for which little information is available on their constituents, can increase the risk of adverse reactions, particularly in pregnant women (Ozioma and Chinwe, 2019). Currently, there is not enough information to recommend the safe use of herbal medicinal products during pregnancy, as most herbal remedies used across sub-Saharan Africa are not backed by robust scientific studies. Moreover, several local herbal remedies used by sub-Saharan African pregnant women have never been botanically identified (Hajj and Holst, 2020). There are also other substances that are used which are not plant based and are commonly used. For example, a common native product eaten by West African women to reduce nausea and vomiting and over salivation is Calabash chalk which is imported to Western countries. Calabash chalk contains high concentrations of lead and has been found to cause gastrointestinal disorders (Moses et al., 2012).

MEDICINE USE IN PREGNANCY IN THE MIDDLE EAST

The cultural views of medicine use in pregnancy in Arabian cultures means that beneficial treatment may be avoided despite being advised by a medical practitioner. The use of common herbs such as peppermint, ginger, thyme, chamomile, sage, aniseed, fenugreek and green tea has been found to be a common practice in the Middle East during pregnancy (John and Shantakumari, 2015). Pain killers and antibiotics are products believed to be harmful during pregnancy (Aljoher et al., 2018). A cultural belief is that using herbal medicines in pregnancy is safer with less side effects in pregnancy than modern medicine and this information is passed down by the woman's friends and family. In addition, the first trimester is believed to be the critical period in which medications and herbals should be avoided (Aljoher et al., 2018). The conditions that these herbs are used for should be reviewed by the midwife or medical practitioner, as gastrointestinal disorders and cold and flu symptoms can be serious in pregnancy and women should seek medical advise for these ailments rather than using herbal remedies. The majority of Middle Eastern women may use these products during their first trimester and conceal this from their medical practitioner (John and Shantakumari, 2015).

CHINESE MEDICINE AND PREGNANCY

Chinese women use traditional medicine for treatment, especially during pregnancy, which has a relatively high usage rate. In addition, for most traditional Chinese medicines there are no instructions for pregnant women or the foetus (Chen et al., 2015). Some of the medicines which are commonly used during pregnancy contain ingredients such as radix bupleuri, coptis (a plant) which could cause uterine contractions and can even lead to abortion (Chen et al., 2015). However, Chinese herbal medicines have been used to prevent spontaneous abortion and preterm labour, and to manage the common cold, low back pain, placenta praevia and foetal growth. In traditional Chinese medicine the body and mind are believed to be inseparable, therefore anything that influences a woman's mind or spirit affects the heart and can affect the foetus in the uterus (Lau, 2012). Therefore, traditional medicine may be used to restore physical and emotional harmony.

However, due to preference for traditional medicine, avoidance of modern medicine may lead to adverse outcomes for women.

SOUTH ASIAN MEDICINE USE DURING PREGNANCY

In South Asian cultures medicines are commonly used in medicinal baths, enemas or as ointments to treat nausea during pregnancy or to stimulate labour (De Boer and Cotington, 2014; Withers et al., 2018). Herbal oral medicines are used by women to treat a number of reproductive health problems, including any discomfort or dysfunctions of pregnancy and labour (Beal, 1998). Plants have also been reported to be used as abortifacients, contraceptives, to stimulate breast milk and to contract the uterus in the post period (Van Andel et al., 2014; De Boer and Cotington, 2014). It is also essential to note that most South Asian women consider herbs and remedies derived from plants to be safer than pharmaceutical drugs.

CARIBBEAN TRADITIONAL MEDICINE AND PREGNANCY

Traditional healing is widely used in Caribbean populations (McKenzie et al., 2011). This is mostly as a result of ancestry from African and East Indian cultures. There are three main systems of healing: 'Bush' or folk medicine, magical religious or spiritual medicine and balance in food and nutrition (McKenzie et al., 2011). Traditionally, flora growing throughout the Caribbean has been used to treat a variety of ailments from colds and flus to more intense issues like infections and parasites (Billcock, 2019).

Practice Point

It is important to note that native herbs and remedies that women may use in pregnancy are imported and can be found in Western countries. At the booking interview a discussion on medicine use with the woman is important and should be undertaken. However, a midwife should be mindful that women from different cultures may be using traditional or alternative medicines. Seeking out this information is an essential task so that appropriate advice can be provided.

The recommended practice in Western cultures is that women are advised to seek medical advice before taking medication in pregnancy; this should be reiterated throughout the woman's care. However, there may be issues in some cultures where medication use in pregnancy is avoided, and a woman could be advised to take medication by a healthcare professional. Awareness of the beliefs that women may have about use of medicines during pregnancy is important. Respecting cultural beliefs around medicine use is also crucial and sensitive discussions should be undertaken to dispel any myths.

Traditional Practices During Labour

BIRTH COMPANIONS

It is noted that most of the traditional beliefs and practices in different cultures are not harmful to women or their babies. In fact, many could have psychological and physical benefits for women, such as confinement practices (Withers et al., 2018). Therefore, midwives should recognise and appreciate these widespread practices when both promoting and providing care. Women from societies where men are traditionally the decision makers may be closely attended by their husbands during pregnancy and childbirth and the husband may often speak for his wife (Dean, 2010). If this is the case then the midwife should always ensure opportunities for the woman to ask and answer questions. In other cultures men are forbidden to enter the labour room or will need to attend accompanied by another female. For example, in Judaism the husband is simply not permitted to watch the birth unless absolutely necessary as the woman is considered to be in an unpure state (Wehbe-Alamah et al., 2021). During labour, the Jewish husband cannot touch or provide any physical support for his wife, nor can he look at any uncovered parts of her body and usually remains at the head of the bed, facing away from the birth (Noble et al., 2009). The mother therefore receives support from a female family member who can act as a doula. Also, in Judaism, *negiah* (touch) is a rule in Jewish law that forbids contact with members of the opposite sex except for spouse, children, grandchildren, parents and grandparents (Kaplan, 2004).

This practice is also common where presence of men is prohibited or not recommended due to risk of harm. For example, during labour Hispanics maintain the traditional cultural belief that having the father view the mother or baby during the birth may be injurious to one or both of them (Darby, 2007). In the Caribbean, fathers in the delivery room are rare, with men being denied access by staff (Ocho et al., 2018). However, women from other cultures may also prefer to be attended by their mothers or other female family members and not have men in the room because of concerns about modesty. These concerns are often raised with women from the Muslim culture with modesty as an important value linked to religion (Dean, 2010). The midwife should be aware of this. At times it is easily demonstrated by the woman wearing clothing that covers the body and head so the female body is not exposed. There is likelihood of women who have concerns about modesty and privacy to be concerned about touch. This is always an issue the midwife should consider. Hence, clear explanation about any procedures that involve touch such as abdominal palpation and vaginal examinations is crucial.

Practice Point

The myriad of birth companion practices in different cultures makes it difficult for the midwife to determine what each woman prefers; therefore, sensitivity is needed to ensure cultural preferences are respected. Other women may view physical contact with members of the opposite gender as unacceptable regardless of their religion or culture and may request same gender healthcare providers and require accommodations to preserve their modesty and dignity. Prohibitions against viewing the female body in some cultures may require that the woman will request that midwives and any other health professionals are also women (Lauderdale, 2008). A culturally sensitive approach is for the midwife to respect and protect these preferences and accommodate the women's wishes as much as possible (Dean, 2010). Midwives should be aware of these different cultural practices and discuss this with the woman during the antenatal period or when devising a birth plan.

LABOUR PRACTICES

Intrapartum practice will vary in different cultures and there are stark differences between Western and non-Western cultures. Typically care in labour in Western cultures occurs in a techno centric environment with close monitoring for mother and baby, the woman often on a bed and input from the medical team. In non-Western cultures birth is typically allowed to progress with women in upright positions supported by family members, typically female and encouragement to eat and drink.

Migrant women have expressed their preference of giving birth naturally (Higginbottom et al., 2013). There are many cultural misconceptions around the course of obstructed or prolonged labour. This makes it difficult to provide information that the woman and her family are willing to accept. For example, in Asian cultures prolonged and obstructed labour are perceived to be a modern-day event due to a sedentary lifestyle (Mirzabagi et al., 2013). Myths such as makes it difficult to educate women on the causes of a delay in their labour. Obstetric intervention is also feared in Asian culture as the stigma of having surgery or an episiotomy was regarded as an inability to perform the role expected of women (Withers et al., 2018). However, some cultural practices are beneficial and are recommended in all maternity settings. For example, Asian women traditionally prefer birthing positions such as squatting, kneeling and sitting (Morrison et al., 2014; Culhane-Pera et al., 2015). These practices are evidenced based and should be facilitated by the midwife for all women in appropriate situations.

Among African women, there is also a strong stigma attached to caesarean births that extends to denigrating the woman to 'a less complete woman' (Adeoye and Kalu, 2011). Hence, women who have this cultural perception that vaginal birth should be achieved to confirm womanhood may avoid procedures such as induction of labour or decline caesarean section if medically recommended. All of these factors can lead to a woman not engaging with maternity care. In some cases a woman may not attend for a post-date appointment due to fear of being offered an induction of labour. Awareness of these issues can enable the midwife to have sensitive discussions with women about prolonged pregnancy and possible interventions during labour. An appropriate discussion by the midwife with the woman can provide a platform to dispel any myths and encourage cultural practices that are beneficial to the woman during labour.

CULTURAL PERCEPTIONS OF LABOUR PAIN

Childbirth is a unique experience for each woman. How she perceives and makes meaning of her pain, as well as her pain-related behaviours while giving birth, are culturally defined (Callister et al., 2003). A dominant narrative across geographical regions is the expectation that silent endurance of pain was part of the role of women as mothers, their reproductive responsibility for ensuring safe childbirth and healthy children (Raman et al., 2016). In their study of pain in childbirth, Callister et al. (2003) found that pain-related behaviours varied among cultural groups, Muslim women tended to be more verbally expressive, Chinese women reported that it was shameful to scream and that it used up the energy that would be needed for the baby's delivery and Mayan women from Guatemala tended to accept pain as an obligation and to approach labour with stoic dignity (Callister et al., 2003).

Verbal expressions of pain and imploring prayers to Allah are common behaviours of Muslim women during labour. It is believed by some women that the louder and more obvious the suffering, the more considerate the husband will be during the postpartum period (Weber, 1996). European and American women are said to show a wide range of reactions to labour pain (Du Gas, 1983) and therefore expression of pain can be very individual to the woman. In some societies childbirth pain has been accepted as a part of women's life and considered a fundamental element for spiritual development. For example, childbirth for African women is viewed as a spiritual journey to gaining self-worth and hope (Bassey Etowa, 2012). In Nigeria, cultural prejudice accounts for inadequate demand for labour pain relief (Obuna and Umeora, 2014). In some Ghanaian cultural groups, there is a belief that it is humiliating if others know one cannot bear labour pain. As a result, women who are unable to endure labour pain are labelled as emotionally weak (Aziato et al., 2016). Caribbean women's expressions of pain during labour are linked to their African ancestry, so similar perceptions of labour pain and expression may be observed.

Migrant women usually prefer the use of other more traditional methods to relieve pain such as walking or drinking hot or cold tea (Murray et al., 2010). Some women view pain as a necessary part of the birth process and satisfaction with the birth experience is more often associated with the sense of fulfilment than with the absence of pain (Callister et al., 2003). Midwives can become culturally sensitive when they understand that responses to pain differ in women according to their cultural norms. It is important to note that these cultural responses to pain are very individual and what is required is the midwife to not make assumptions about what pain relief is required by the woman during pregnancy and childbirth.

Practice Point

Offering pain relief to women should not be done on a routine basis or based on a preconceived idea of pain tolerance in women from different cultures. In fact allowing the woman to request pain relief in the first instance is a more culturally sensitive approach. A woman appearing to be in pain does not necessarily mean she requires pain relief or is not coping is a common misconception from the midwives. Often midwives will base the woman's demonstration of pain on their own personal cultural norm of pain expression which is inappropriate and not culturally safe. This leads to inappropriate discussions around pain relief.

Postpartum Practices for the Mother

PERIOD OF REST

Postpartum practices in Western cultures do not typically extend beyond the first few days postpartum in contrast to many cultures of East Asia, South Asia and the Middle East, which emphasise the practice of social support rituals for a more protracted postpartum period (Posmontier and Horowitz, 2004; Dennis et al., 2007). Traditional postpartum practices persist in many Asian cultures based on the belief that they assure the health of the mother and baby, with failure to comply widely believed to result in long-lasting health problems for both (Syed et al., 2008; Callister et al., 2011). Women in China, Cambodia, Laos, Nepal, Thailand, Myanmar, Singapore and Vietnam similarly believe that the first few days up to 40 days postpartum is a time for isolation and confinement (Syed et al., 2008; Naser et al., 2012). Similar aspects are found in several countries worldwide concerning resting the mother in the postnatal period. The existence of postpartum practices has also been noted in Southeast Asia, South America and Africa (Chou, 2017).

Across 20 countries, each culture's postpartum practice includes a specified rest period, a prescribed diet and organised support from family members (Chou, 2017). The same practices can be found in some Western cultures. In Eastern Europe, women are secluded for the first month after birth. In addition to secluded rest, postpartum body massage and abdominal binding are common throughout Latin America (Major, 2020). African practices include performance of postnatal rituals with herbs, and application of concoctions to prevent postnatal complications (Fantaye et al., 2019). The practice of support is also present in Caribbean cultures where the mother is supported by a female relative who helps with cooking, cleaning and caring for mother and baby. In the Jewish culture, new mothers are required to rest for the first 7 days and are cared for by family members since she is considered to be 'a choleh she' yesh bo sakkannah' (a sick person in danger): family support will last for 6 weeks, promoting maternal rest and recovery (Semenic, 2004).

In contrast, 'for many women in the United States, the 6-week postpartum visit is a period devoid of formal or informal maternal support' (American College of Obstetricians and Gynecologists (ACOG) 2018). This is likely to lead to women being depressed, feeling lonely and unsupported after having a baby. There are issues of stigma and taboo surrounding mental health issues in many cultures prompting rejection by the community (Benza and Liamputtong, 2014). Migrant women may feel stressed from the pressures of having a baby in another country and may hide their feelings. The midwife should be aware of the challenges that women may face in the postnatal period around feeling anxious or depressed by being fearful of seeking help or divulging that they are not coping. Postnatal depression and the harm which might affect the baby has been difficult to understand by some migrant women and there are issues of stigma and taboo leading to women hiding any symptoms (Hill et al., 2012). Therefore, the support provided to new mothers in some cultures should be seen by the midwife as beneficial and a practice that should be continued and supported.

POSTNATAL RITUALS

Postnatal practices in many cultures include aspects of rituals to facilitate the mother returning to pre-pregnancy health. According to the theory of hot/cold foods practised in some cultures, good health requires balancing intake of substances that are hot or cold (Darby, 2007). Because childbirth involves loss of blood, which is hot, the postpartum period is considered cold and the mother requires hot food and a warm environment. There are specific bathing restrictions or prohibitions related to the 'hot' and 'cold' beliefs already discussed. Cold baths or showers are often strictly prohibited to avoid blood clots, sore bones and joints and an itchy body (Dennis et al., 2007) A related practice found among Asian cultures is to actively warm the new mother to balance the loss of 'hot' blood during delivery (Dennis et al., 2007).

Asian cultures practise postpartum massage with oils infused with 'warming' spices, and abdominal binding. This practice is also found in parts of Africa. The physical act of massaging and then firmly wrapping the torso begins within hours or days after vaginal birth and can last from a few weeks to a couple of months, depending on the comfort and beliefs of the individual. In some cultures, binding includes wrapping the hips tightly so that all the muscles involved in the birthing process can heal, as well as wrapping from just below the breasts to the top of the thighs. In the Caribbean, the mother may be asked to consume a herbal drink of mauby bark to cleanse the body and a sheet wrapped around her abdomen to aid uterine involution.

The Jewish laws of Niddah is referred to as a state of impurity (DeVito, 2019). Immediately after birth, a woman is considered niddah and must remain sexually separated from her husband for a period of 7 days after the birth of a male child and 14 days after the birth of a female child.

Hygiene rituals in many cultures occur as the postpartum woman is seen as contaminated, and therefore special hygiene practices are required (Rice et al., 1999). This may mean that the mother is unable to leave the house or go to church until she has ceased bleeding. Creative strategies for encouraging hygiene (e.g., sponge baths, perineal care), exercise and nutritional balance will be needed while remaining respectful of the cultural significance of the practices (Dean, 2010).

Dennis et al. (2007) in a literature review concluded that healthcare providers should consider the major similarities between cultural postpartum practices to deliver culturally competent peri-natal care. These practices should be encouraged and provide psychological support to the mother. What the midwife should be cognisant of are dangerous practices such as using heat to reduce the amount of blood loss after birth or the drinking of herbal remedies that may be contraindicated for breastfeeding. Midwives who work with postpartum women will benefit from understanding beliefs that underpin these practices.

PLACENTA PRACTICES

Many cultural ideas regarding the placenta involve beliefs that indicate that the specific means of treatment/disposal can affect some aspect of a person's life, usually the mother or the child. This is found in African, Asian and some European cultures (Young and Benyshek, 2010). Rituals for the placenta may include wrapping in certain fabrics or plants, placing in a specific vessel and burying in a particular location. For example, African practices include retrieval and burial of the placenta, often around the woman's home (Fantaye et al., 2019). In Jamaica, although the placenta is buried, it is the burial of the umbilical cord or navel string that attracts ritualistic behaviour (Tortello, 2021). This cord is buried in a special location and a tree is planted on that spot, usually a coconut or a breadfruit tree which becomes known as a birth tree, which symbolises a spiritual attachment to a place.

Practice Point

Postpartum practices include culturally influenced behavioural adjustments that women and their families follow during the postpartum period to help the woman recover from giving birth. Family members offer practical, social and emotional assistance as the woman follows dietary adjustments and hygiene practices for a specific amount of time, usually 3 to 5 weeks. In many ways the midwife should see some postnatal practice as being beneficial for the woman – the resting, being fed and family support. However, the mother should be educated on seeking healthcare for herself and her baby if there are any signs of ill health, as she may delay leaving her home due to wishing to adhere to the lying-in period or 40-day rule.

Postpartum Practices for the Baby
EARLY BATHING

There are cultural beliefs related to early newborn bathing. The World Health Organization (WHO, 2013) released recommendations to delay the first bath until 24 hours after birth. If there are cultural reasons, bathing should be delayed at least 6 hours after birth to allow the neonate to transition to extrauterine life, therefore supporting bonding and early breastfeeding. In Asian cultures it is believed that early bathing should be done to remove the dirty coating of vernix, to clean and purify the baby (Memon et al., 2019). In some African cultures, the main reason for the universal early bathing, including at health facilities, was a belief that the birth fluids caused body odour later in life; the vernix is described as being dirty and linked to poor maternal dietary behaviour (Adejuyigbe et al., 2015). For example, in Nigeria, the vernix is removed immediately with oil and bathing. However, in Tanzania and Ethiopia, the vernix may be removed by just wiping. Subsequent bathing was also done frequently in African cultures, where newborns were bathed between two and five times a day and frequent bathing is the cultural norm. Key themes were that bathing was essential for health, important to keep the baby clean, fresh and sweat free and to help them feel comfortable, sleep and grow (Adejuyigbe et al., 2015).

In the Middle East, the practice of salting the baby is common. This involves rubbing the baby with salt in a small amount of water. Reported reasons for adopting this practice include prevention of bad odours from sweating; protecting skin from different disorders during childhood, such as skin redness, infection and nappy rash; and protecting skin from dryness during the lifetime (Abuidhail, 2014). The process of salting may be continued up until 40 days.

INFANT MASSAGE

Infant massage is common in non-Western cultures and is becoming more popular in Western countries. Baby massage is widely practised in Indian and other Asian settings and is commonly performed by mothers or other family members using oil (Chaturvedi et al., 2017). The benefits of massage on the baby are believed to improve skin integrity and digestion. The traditional practice of oil massage in India has its roots in the ancient traditional medicine of Ayurveda. The Ayurvedic literature recommends oil massage to infants until 1 year to promote healthy development (Tewari, 1997). The same practices are also used in Arab societies where the use of oils in massages is used to test ill health in newborns (Arabiat et al., 2019). Also prevalent in Arabian cultures is swaddling newborns by tightly wrapping the legs straight and binding both arms by the side of the newborn's trunk, performed to generally strengthen the newborn's muscles and to prevent any injury when carrying the newborn (Arabiat et al., 2019). This practice is believed by mothers to be essential for baby's well-being.

In African cultures, baby massage is also common. Emollient application in the first months of life is a normative, long-standing tradition in some African countries. Emollients are applied for various reasons including to make the skin 'soft', 'smooth', 'attractive', 'healthy', 'strong' and 'rash free', to keep the baby warm (all sites), to soften/strengthen the joints/bones, shape the baby, ensure flexibility and encourage growth and weight gain (Amare et al., 2015). In addition, babies are kept close to mother by the carrying of the baby on the mother's back (Worthman et al., 2010). This is to provide comfort to the baby and allow the mother to continue with her chores. In the Caribbean, massage of the baby to stretch the limbs using coconut oil is performed and the baby wears amulets to ward off the evil eye.

CORD CARE IN DIFFERENT CULTURES

Cord care practices vary by cultural groups within a country and employ a wide range of substances led by a desire to promote healing and hasten cord separation (Coffey and Brown, 2017). Hence, there are various underlying beliefs related to application of substances to the umbilical cord. Other beliefs related to cord care practices are performed to keep evil spirits away and prevent pain and bleeding. Potentially harmful cord care cultural practices predominate in parts of sub-Saharan Africa (Sacks et al., 2015; Semrau et al., 2016). African practices that are deemed harmful include clamping the baby's umbilical cord and applying charcoal powder and herbal extract powders made of roots, burnt gourds or ash, petroleum jelly, commercial baby lotion, cooking oil and breast milk to the cord stump (Sacks et al., 2015; Fantaye et al., 2019).

Substances are also used on the cord in Caribbean cultures. For example, in Jamaica nutmeg may be used to dress the baby's cord (Tortello, 2021).

Similar harmful practices are also seen in Arabian/Middle Eastern societies where ethanol, antibiotic powder or coffee grounds are applied to the cord (Arabiat et al., 2019). In Turkey, cord care practices include putting substances in the cord to make it dry and separate faster, tying the baby's abdomen and using a butter cloth for infected cords (Alparslan and Demirel, 2013). In Jordan, neomycin powder is used or Kohla (a handmade mixture of ground lead with the powdered stones of olives or dates) is applied to the cord.

There are also reports of using traditional substances on the cord in Asian cultures (Memon et al., 2019). In Asian cultures there is a variety of cord care practices that are harmful. In India herbal paste or mustard oil is applied to umbilical cords (Ghosh and Sharma, 2010) and in Pakistan ointment, ghee, coconut oil and mustard oil are applied. Some also applied surma (locally made kohl), clove oil, turmeric and talcum powder (Ayaz and Saleem, 2010; Gul et al., 2014). In China there is a belief that keeping the cord uncovered will allow cold air to enter the baby and cause illness and substances are used to heal the cord (Xu et al., 2018).

Exercise

Review the following scenario:

A midwife attends Sabine for a home postnatal check at 5 days after birth. On performing the postnatal check, the midwife notices that Sabine is using herbs and heat to treat the baby's umbilical cord.

1. How can the midwife support safe cultural practices and advise on unsafe practices in a culturally sensitive way?
2. What is the key information the midwife should provide to Sabine?

Practice Point

The midwife has an important role in ensuring mothers are not using harmful practice for cord care. A discussion with the mother about appropriate cord care should be undertaken so that she can be educated on how to care effectively for her baby's cord. It may be beneficial to inform the mother of any knowledge of harmful cord care practices that different cultures may use and acknowledge understanding of cultural tradition. This approach further opens up the discussion and may prompt the mother to discuss her cultural practices on cord care.

BREASTFEEDING

There are specific cultural practices related to breastfeeding. Many African and Asian communities share the mistaken belief that breastfeeding should be delayed for several days after birth, and that colostrum should not be fed to newborn babies (Adamson, 2015). There is a belief that colostrum is dirty is found in African cultures and it was believed to be also useful for cleansing the babies the infants intestines or that breast milk that's sits in the breast for more than 2 hours is old (Steinman et al., 2010; Textor et al., 2013; Gallegos et al., 2015). Giving a mixture of boiled water, sugar and salt to babies to cleanse their stomachs to ease digestion and boost immunity is performed in some African cultures (Sacks et al., 2015). African immigrant mothers maintain infant feeding practices from their countries of origin such as eating of special foods to aid milk production and enhance breastfeeding, but they also adopted some of the practices of the host country such as not breastfeeding in public places, which is contrary to practices in their home country (Gallegos et al., 2015). In some Caribbean women it is generally the family that influences the woman's decision to breastfeed and how much support is given (Ingram et al., 2008).

In certain Hindus, female family members symbolically wash the mother's breasts prior to the initiation of breastfeeding (Gatrad et al., 2004). Giving infants honey or grounded, filtered sugar before beginning breastfeeding is found in Asian cultures. The belief is that it cleans the intestine and makes it soft so the infant can pass meconium easily (Fatmi et al., 2005). Bangladeshi and Pakistani grandmothers are known to give all babies small amounts of boiled water from a few days old, however, Indian grandmothers suggested the same practice from a few weeks old (Ingram et al., 2003). Their thinking is that if a baby is thirsty their skin will be dry but not if they drink water. The beliefs of grandmothers are transmitted to younger generations of mothers and are followed (Ingram et al., 2003).

In Arabian cultures, breastfeeding is valued, however, there are beliefs around insufficient milk or milk being impure. This is one of the main reasons given by mothers for giving up exclusive breastfeeding or delaying breastfeeding and giving newborns honey and fenugreek (herbaceous plant of the pea family) at the first feed or anise and water (Arabiat et al., 2019). Giving these products to the newborn is believed to cleanse the stomach and import immunity and well-being.

In orthodox Jewish women, although breastfeeding is allowed, mechanical breast pumps may not be used on the Sabbath as this is seen as work. Women may hand express the milk, as long as it is expressed either over the sink or into a salt-laden container so that it may not be used (Chertok, 1999). In most parts of Africa most participants' personal accounts revealed the use of prelacteal fluid and food before the initiation of breastfeeding, which could sometimes continue until 4 days after birth, irrespective of whether it was the first or subsequent deliveries (Joseph and Earland, 2019).

The consumption of a special postpartum diet has been traditionally regarded as beneficial to breast milk quantity and quality. Such cultural belief is still prevalent among Chinese mothers living in China and abroad in recent decades (Zhou et al., 2010).

Exercise

Review the following scenario:

A midwife discovers a mother giving her 1-day-old baby fluids. On questioning, the mother explains that she is waiting for her milk to come in as she does not want to give the baby colostrum.

1. What questions should the midwife ask the mother?
2. How could the midwife support and advise the mother whilst remaining culturally sensitive?

Practice Point

The midwife has an important role in educating mothers about the benefits of breastfeeding. This should be done in a culturally sensitive way. A discussion must include the potential harm that can be caused by giving the baby anything else but breast milk. However, acknowledgement of the mother's cultural beliefs and the influence of family and friends is important.

NAMING CEREMONIES

Naming ceremonies where the newborn baby is officially given a name vary across different cultures and religions. Usually, the ceremony is attended by family and friends and includes a celebration involving prayers and food.

Muslims name their children within 7 days of birth and do so on the advice of the Hadith. Within 7 days, a ceremony known as an 'Aqiqah' is held to thank God or Allah (Gatrad et al., 2004). The baby's head is shaved and there is a feast for friends and family in celebration, and, usually, a goat is sacrificed with the meat being distributed (Choudhary et al., 2017).

In Judaism, Islam and Hinduism religions this can occur from the 7th to 12th day after birth. Jewish baby naming ceremonies are considered to be one of the most important rituals and involve giving the child their Hebrew name, which 'could be a name that sounds like the baby's secular/English name, or it could be a name that is significant to the family' (Tory, 2013). Boys will receive their Hebrew name 8 days after birth; there is no set time for naming girls, but it typically happens within a few weeks of birth.

In Hinduism, a *Namakarana* ceremony is typically performed on the 10th or the 12th day after birth. The naming ceremony may also be done on the first new moon or full moon day after the 10th day of birth (Roya, 2017). There may be consultation of an astrologer for a suitable name for the baby, or an ancestor's name may be chosen or the baby may be named after a favourite Hindu deity.

In China, it is unlucky for a baby to be named before the birth, placing an importance on the naming ceremony. The naming ceremony usually takes place after a month due to the fear of naming a baby who may not survive the neonatal period. Since it is considered unlucky to name a baby before birth, parents use what is called a 'milk name' before a formal given name is chosen. This name is known only by the parents or close family members (Moore, 2007).

In Africa the naming of a child is a mark or expression of authority over the child by the parents and the community into which the child is born. Since the father is the head of the family, it is the father that gives the child a name (Kanu, 2019). The naming of a child is also symbolic of the incorporation of the child into the family or community. This is even more obvious in circumstances when the child is given the name of an ancestor of the community or family. The name of a child in African societies can also be monumental to mark an event that has happened in the community and also prophetic to bless the future of a child (Kanu, 2019). In West Africa, it is common for newborns to be given special names based on the day on which they were born. For example, ethnicities in Ghana and surrounding areas have different traditional names which are given to the baby based on the day they are born, with some flexibility.

MALE CIRCUMCISION

Globally, 30% of men undergo circumcision mainly for religious and cultural reasons (Weiss et al., 2007). Circumcision is a religious requirement for all male Muslims as it helps with maintenance of hygiene, ablution and reduction in the incidence of certain health issues such as cervical cancer (in wives of circumcised men) and penile cancer (Rassool, 2014). Two-thirds of male circumcision is in Muslims. Other common determinants of male circumcision are ethnicity, perceived health and sexual benefits and the desire to conform to social norms (WHO, 2007).

The practice of male circumcision for religious or cultural reasons is also found in North America, Africa and Asia. Circumcision has been practised for non-religious reasons for many thousands of years in sub-Saharan Africa, and in many ethnic groups around the world. In the majority of these cultures, circumcision is an integral part of a rite-of-passage to manhood (Wilcken et al., 2010).

In Jewish religion the male infant is traditionally circumcised on the eighth day of life as long as there are no medical contraindications (Semenic et al., 2004). The justification, in the Jewish holy book the Torah, is that a covenant was made between Abraham and God, the outward sign of which is circumcision for all Jewish males. Newborn circumcision is also common in Israel, the United States of America, Canada, Australia and New Zealand (WHO, 2007).

PROTECTION OF THE NEWBORN

Various cultural practice and rituals are performed to protect the newborn; most of these practices are harmless. Therefore, the midwife should be respectful of the woman's wishes. In Hinduism and Buddhism, a small 'Bindi' or mark is put on the middle of the child's forehead in the form of a red powder/paste, as a blessing to the child and a welcome to the world. A Muslim family may wish a male relative to whisper the Islamic call to prayer into the baby's ear and perhaps attach an amulet around the baby's neck or wrist.

Also, some Muslims perform the practices of putting honey in the newborn's mouth or putting a date on the infant's mouth and reciting the Quran before the first feeding of the infant (Yavuz et al., 2020). In Arabian/Middle Eastern cultures the practice of putting an amulet on the newborn in the shape of a hand and Kohl on the baby's eyes is believed to help banish evil or negative energy away from their newborn (Arabiat et al., 2019). In African and Caribbean cultures an open Bible is often placed in a newborn's cot, for protection of the baby and to ward off evil. The Bible is usually left open at a Psalm. In Jamaica, a red string may be tied around a newborn's wrist, or in the hair. This is to chase ghosts away and ward off evil.

It is hoped that this broad overview of different cultural beliefs and norms related to pregnancy and childbirth highlights the diverse context of women's viewpoints. The next sections will discuss other cultures that should be considered by midwives when providing care to women.

Midwives' Professional and Workplace Culture

In this section we will look at the professional and workplace culture of the midwife and how this may differ to the culture of the woman. This is an important consideration as we have already talked about women having different cultures and how this may be conveyed in social interactions. However, in addition to having a personal culture, the midwife will also have a professional culture that she adheres to. The dynamics of these two cultures are significant as there will be challenges for the midwife when providing care to women.

ENCULTURATION IN MIDWIFERY PRACTICE

The midwifery profession has developed a culture with norms and beliefs guided by the statutory framework of their regulatory body. Enculturation is the process whereby individuals learn their group's culture through experience, observation and instruction (Gavelek and Kong, 2012). This is different to acculturation discussed in Chapter 1, which occurs when a newcomer is not a member of the community they have migrated into. In enculturation the newcomer is normally an immature member of a community (Kirshner and Meng, 2012). This can be likened to a student midwife entering the profession of midwifery. A professional code of conduct stipulates how a midwife should act in order to maintain the integrity of the profession (NMC, 2018). Hence, professional culture may be conformed to despite the midwife's own individual cultural beliefs. It is suggested that many midwives have also been socialised into assuming control as part of their role as a health professional and may fail to identify and legitimise the cultural identity of the women they care for (Phiri et al., 2010). Midwifery culture may be internalised by individuals entering the profession created by training and teaching methods, which individuals adopt to in order to become part of the profession (Arundell et al., 2018). So, conflicts can occur if the professional culture of midwifery contradicts the personal culture of the midwife. The dilemma that a midwife may face if this situation occurs can impact on the care provided to the woman. This will be even more so if the culture of the woman is totally disregarded and deemed to be unimportant resulting in ethnocentrism.

THE IMPACT OF ETHNOCENTRISM

It is alleged that healthcare professionals tend to lean towards ethnocentrism (Giger and Davidhizar, 2002; Capell et al., 2008; Jordal and Wahlberg, 2018; Markey et al., 2018). Ethnocentrism commonly refers to the tendency to view the world through the lens of one's own culture. This perspective generally creates feelings of cultural superiority resulting in justification of prejudicial treatment of outsider groups (Sefiha, 2007). It is believed that everyone is ethnocentric and it is human nature to believe that your cultural beliefs and values are better that others. Midwives are not immune from this fact however, as already discussed the conflict between the personal culture of the midwife and the professional culture are two things that may impact on the woman's culture. Ethnocentrism can lead to discrimination against people who are different and can impact in the midwife's providing culturally competent care (Capell et al., 2008). Issues of racism, prejudice and stereotyping are also related to ethnocentrism.

Midwives who study other cultures attempt to limit ethnocentric thinking by practising cultural relativity which involves judging other groups by their own cultural standards and their own point of view (Sefiha, 2007). It is said that cultural relativism is the opposite of ethnocentrism. Cultural relativity critics argue that cultural relativism discourages cross-cultural criticism, rejects universal morality and sanctions human-rights abuses and terrorism (Brown, 2004).

ELEMENTS OF WORKPLACE CULTURE

Workplace culture is comprised of four elements: artefacts, behavioural norms, values and assumptions (Davis and Homer, 2016). Artefacts include symbols and objects that express cultural messages. In the maternity context these might include the equipment or signage visible in a birthing room or the way a room is set up in expectation of a particular type of birth. The second element concerns the overarching culture of an organisation, including consistent practices, beliefs and attitudes in a maternity unit (Wagner et al., 2014). Behavioural norms are the behaviours and practices that are expected and 'allowed' within a workplace; values are not always those articulated in advertising materials but are most clearly illustrated by the practices, outcomes and priorities encouraged and rewarded by a workplace (Davis and Homer, 2016). If there are particular ways of performing or behaving in a workplace, this may become an integral part of a midwife's beliefs and attitudes. While an organisation might state that they value woman-centred care they may in fact prioritise and encourage efficiency. Finally, assumptions are the beliefs that underpin all other aspects of workplace culture. In the maternity setting, assumptions may include that birth is inherently risky or that all women will require pain relief in labour (Braithwaite et al., 2017).

IMPACT OF WORKPLACE CULTURE ON MIDWIFERY PRACTICE

The workplace environment also has influences on the midwife's behaviour and views and is important to sustaining and retaining the midwifery workforce. Workplace culture affects midwives' professional practice, including their ability to 'be with' women (Davis and Homer, 2016). New staff are socialised into workplace culture, either explicitly or indirectly, learning how things are done and what is expected. Often, the culture of a workplace can be 'felt' by the employees who work there and by the consumers using the service (Schein, 2010). It may also influence midwifery students' clinical learning and their attitudes towards the profession (Arundell et al., 2018). The culture of the maternity unit is also influential in delivering care that is women-centred, clinically effective and continually improving in response to a changing context. There has been increasing attention on culture in healthcare, particularly organisational and corporate cultures, rather than the immediate culture experienced by patients and users at the interface of care – the microsystems level which we term 'workplace culture' (Manley et al., 2011). Without concerted efforts to explore, understand and challenge the interplay of overt and covert beliefs at work within organisational cultures, counterproductive biases and behaviours can persist. Many public health professionals recognise that failing to consider the cultural contexts of their professional actions can impede their ability to improve working practices, and to identify productive innovations and scale them up (WHO, 2017).

IMPACT OF OTHER PROFESSIONALS' CULTURE ON MIDWIFERY PRACTICE

There might be ideas about appropriate professional roles and delineations; expectations about patients' and carers' knowledge and dispositions; and assumptions about the relative power of healthcare professionals – collectively and individually – in the health system (Mannion and Davies, 2018).

This might include prevailing views on patient needs, autonomy and dignity; ideas about evidence for action; and expectations about safety, quality, clinical performance and service improvement (Schein, 2010). Studies examining midwifery practice in hospital settings suggest that powerful cultural norms shape practice in these settings (O'Connell and Downe, 2009).

Within healthcare, taking an organisational culture perspective means accepting that care and caring practices are influenced by contextual structures such as political, economic, technical and legal dimensions (Rytterström et al., 2009). According to Rytterstörm et al. (2009) these dimensions create dominant values, norms and beliefs that shape how individuals give meaning to their tasks and how care is practised.

Providing Transcultural Midwifery Care

CULTURAL COMPETENCY IN MIDWIFERY PRACTICE

In a previous chapter we talked about the components of cultural competency and their importance in midwifery practice. Cultural competence means both recognising the impact of your own culture and beliefs on your midwifery practice and being able to acknowledge and incorporate each woman's cultures into the provision of individualised midwifery care. It means having the knowledge, skills and attitudes to understand the effect of power within a healthcare relationship and to develop respectful relationships with people of different cultures (Durie, 2001). In the next section we will talk about cultural safety, but cultural knowledge, sensitivity and awareness are some requisites that can be useful in caring for women. Cultural values and perceptions that health professionals hold are important to examine because they may serve as a lens through which clients' needs are interpreted; there are times when the caregiver thinks she or he understands but may have misinterpreted because of her/his own unexamined cultural filters (Kang, 2014). Value of nonjudgmental support for women's cultural practices can be in conflict with the value of scientific/evidence-based practice when working with women whose cultural practices may be at odds with what the healthcare professionals consider to be evidence-based practice (Kang, 2014). Cultural self-awareness is paramount to intercultural practice because being acutely aware of the influence of one's cultural values and beliefs can help midwives avoid demoting other values and beliefs and become more conscious of the dynamics of power when providing care (Hays, 2008).

In order to ensure that care is culturally sensitive the woman's needs and expectations need to be met as far as possible. It is unreasonable for migrant women to expect the UK healthcare system to cater to all their cultural needs. However, there should be respect, compromise and acknowledgement from healthcare professionals of these cultural needs. Cultural knowledge should be used as a springboard in order to overcome any misconceptions (Esegbona-Adeigbe, 2011). Asking questions about a woman's culture will demonstrate a midwife's interest and will facilitate greater understanding of the woman's needs. Questions may be specific or general depending on the circumstances. Look at the next exercise with some examples of questions, which may be beneficial for a midwife to ask women.

Exercise

The following questions can be utilised by midwives to begin to explore cultural practice with women:
1. What foods do you commonly eat?
2. Is the gender of the healthcare professional important to you?
3. Who do you expect to be with you during the birth of your baby?
4. Are there any birth rituals that need to be performed for you and the baby?
5. In your culture do you give colostrum to your baby?
6. Who cares for the mother after the birth of the baby?

Asking questions can reveal indirect information that can be used to provide individualised care. Often midwives may use the same approach to care for every woman which may not be appropriate in some cases. Being exposed to differences between the woman's culture and the midwife's culture increases critical consciousness which will be discussed at the end of this chapter.

USING CULTURAL COMPETENCY MODEL IN MIDWIFERY PRACTICE

CASE 4.1 CULTURAL COMPETENCY MODEL

A case study of a midwife using the cultural competency model to facilitate her practice.
Hannah is a midwife working in a busy maternity unit that has a high number of migrant women using the services.

Cultural awareness – Hannah is aware that normal practice in the UK may be different to the women that she cares for. Hannah undertakes a reflective exercise to explore how she has acquired her personal and professional beliefs on pregnancy care and how women may acquire their own culture.

Cultural sensitivity – Hannah has become aware of cultural differences through personal reflection. Now that she is aware of these differences she has become more sensitive to women's cultural values by respecting individual women's wishes and considering their cultural needs when providing care.

Cultural knowledge – Hannah realises that women from a particular culture regularly attend her maternity unit. Hence, she has gained knowledge of particular rituals and norms practised in this culture. Hannah is aware that culture is very individual and so at every opportunity will ask a woman if she practices a ritual or norm common in her culture so that she can adjust the care she provides to accommodate this.

Cultural encounters – Hannah has regular contact with women from different cultures and is now beginning to build a knowledge base of cultures that she has frequent contact with.

Cultural desire – There are some cultures that Hannah only has contact with on a limited basis. However, if an opportunity arises to care for a woman from a different culture, she takes the opportunity and is confident in interacting with her and her family.

Cultural competency – Hannah regularly adapts her practice to meet the cultural needs of any women she provides care for and takes the opportunity to empower women.

APPLICATION OF CULTURAL SAFETY IN PRACTICE

In Chapter 1 the importance of cultural safety was discussed, along with the need for the midwife to be aware of power imbalances that may occur between health professionals and the woman. In addition, the need for critical self-awareness of any assumptions and beliefs that the midwife may have that may conflict with the woman's belief was discussed (Curtis et al., 2019). Finally, the understanding that it is the woman who determines that her care is culturally safe is an important concept in cultural safety (Parisa et al., 2016). Therefore, cultural safety should be the ultimate goal for midwives which can be achieved by using a systematic approach.

The next exercise provides an example of how a midwife can apply cultural safety concepts in practice.

Exercise

Sama is caring for Lee who is from another culture and is asking for advice on what type of antenatal care she can have. Sama utilises the following strategies to facilitate cultural safety.

Power Imbalance

Sama is aware that Lee may feel overwhelmed by engaging with maternity services and feels the midwife knows best. However, Sama wishes to explore with Lee what her views are on pregnancy care, particularly in her own culture. In doing this Sama is attempting to change the power imbalances that can occur between a woman and her midwife.

Critical Consciousness

Sama is also critically aware of how her cultural views may conflict with Lee's and makes a conscious effort to address these during the discussion.

Assessing cultural Safety

Sama is aware that it is important for the woman to assess if her care is culturally safe. Sama addresses this by asking Lee directly how she feels about the care provided. In doing this Lee is given an opportunity to provide feedback which Sama can use to discuss any other further concerns Lee may have.

REFLECTIVE QUESTIONS

1. Why is a broad awareness of cultural practice related to childbirth important to midwives?
2. What is your view of cultural practices that are seen to be harmless?
3. How would you facilitate increasing your knowledge on cultural practices and beliefs in pregnancy?
4. How often do you believe critical consciousness should be undertaken in your midwifery practice?

References

Abdullahi, A.A., 2011. Trends and challenges of traditional medicine in Africa. Afr. J. Tradit. Complement. Altern. Med, 8 (5 Suppl), 115–123.

Abuidhail, J., 2014. Rural jordanian mothers' beliefs, knowledge and practices of postnatal care. Qual. Prim. Care. 22 (6), 285–293.

ACOG, 2018. Optimizing postpartum care committee opinion: number 736. Available at: https://www.acog.org/clinical/clinical-guidance/committee-opinion/articles/2018/05/optimizing-postpartum-care.

Adamson, D.S., 2015. The myths about food and pregnancy. https://www.bbc.co.uk/news/magazine-32033409

Adejuyigbe, E.A., Bee, M.H., Amare, Y., Omotara, B.A., Iganus, R.B., Manzi, F., et al., 2015. 'Why not bathe the baby today?': A qualitative study of thermal care beliefs and practices in four African sites. BMC Pediatr. 15 (1), 1–7.

Adeoye, S., Kalu, C.A., 2011. Pregnant Nigerian women's view of caesarean section. Niger. J. Clin. Pract. 14 (3), 276–279.

Agus, Y., Horiuchi, S., Porter, S.E., 2012. Rural Indonesia women's traditional beliefs about antenatal care. BMC Res Notes. 5 (1), 589.

Aljoher, A.M., Alsaeed, M.A., AlKhlfan, M.A., Almethen, A.W., Almukhaitah, M.A., Zareen, H., Alia, S.I., 2018. Pregnant women risk perception of medications and natural products use during pregnancy in Alahsa, Saudi Arabia. Egypt. J. Hosp. Med. 70 (1), 13–20.

Alparslan, Ö., Demirel, Y., 2013. Traditional neonatal care practices in Turkey. Jpn. J. Nurs. Sci 10 (1), 47–54.

Amare, Y., Shamba, D.D., Manzi, F., Bee, M.H., Omotara, B.A., Iganus, R.B., et al., 2015. Current neonatal skin care practices in four African sites. J. Trop. Pediatr. 61 (6), 428–434.

Arabiat, D.H., Whitehead, L., AL Jabery, M., Towell-Barnard, A., Shields, L., Abu Sabah, E., 2019. Traditional methods for managing illness in newborns and infants in an Arab society. Int. Nurs. Rev. 66 (3), 329–337.

Arundell, F., Mannix, J., Sheehan, A., Peters, K., 2018. Workplace culture and the practice experience of midwifery students: a meta-synthesis. J. Nurs. Manag. 26 (3), 302–313.

Ayaz, A., Saleem, S., 2010. Neonatal mortality and prevalence of practices for newborn care in a squatter settlement of Karachi, Pakistan: a cross-sectional study. PloS one 5 (11), e13783.

Aziato, L., Ohene, L.A., Dedey, F., Clegg-Lamptey, J.N.A., 2016. I was in real pain: Surgical nurses' personal pain experiences in Ghana. Int. J. Car. Sci. 9 (1), 90.

Bandyopadhyay, M., 2009. Impact of ritual pollution on lactation and breastfeeding practices in rural West Bengal, India. Int. Breastfeed. J. 4 (2). https://doi.org/10.1186/1746-4358-4-2.

Bassey Etowa, J., 2012. Becoming a mother: the meaning of childbirth for African–Canadian women. Contemp. Nurse 41 (1), 28–40.

Beal, M.W., 1998. Women's use of complementary and alternative therapies in reproductive health care. J. Nurse Midwifery. 43 (3), 224–234.

Benza, S., Liamputtong, P., 2014. Pregnancy, childbirth and motherhood: a meta-synthesis of the lived experiences of immigrant women. Midwifery 30 (6), 575–584.

Billcock, J., 2019. Wild medicine and garden healers. Available at: https://current.seabourn.com/article/wild-medicine-and-garden-healers.

Braithwaite, J., Herkes, J., Ludlow, K., Testa, L., Lamprell, G., 2017. Association between organisational and workplace cultures, and patient outcomes: systematic review. BMJ Open 7, 11.

Brown, D.E., 2004. Human universals, human nature & human culture. Daedalus 133 (4), 47–54.

Callister, L.C., Khalaf, I., Semenic, S., Kartchner, R., Vehvilainen-Julkunen, K., 2003. The pain of childbirth: perceptions of culturally diverse women. Pain Manag. Nurs. 4 (4), 145–154.

Callister, L.C., Khalaf, I., 2010. Spirituality in childbearing women. J. Perinat. Educ. 19 (2), 16–24.

Callister, L.C., Eads, M.N., Diehl, J.P.S.Y., 2011. Perceptions of giving birth and adherence to cultural practices in Chinese women. MCN Am. J. Matern. Child Nurs. 36 (6), 387–394.

Capell, J., Dean, E., Veenstra, G., 2008. The relationship between cultural competence and ethnocentrism of health care professionals. J. Transcult. Nurs. 19 (2), 121–125.

Chakona, G., Shackleton, C., 2019. Food taboos and cultural beliefs influence food choice and dietary preferences among pregnant women in the eastern cape, South Africa. Nutrients. 11 (11), 2668.

Chakrabarti, S., Chakrabarti, A., 2019. Food taboos in pregnancy and early lactation among women living in a rural area of West Bengal. J. Family Med. Prim. Care 8 (1), 86.

Chaturvedi, S., Raven, J., Patwardhan, B., 2017. Addressing child under nutrition: can traditional practices offer a solution? Glob. Health Action. 10 (1), 1327255.

Chen, H.Q., Zou, S.H., Yang, J.B., Cai, J., Zhang, Y., Wang, Z.L., 2015. A survey and analysis of using traditional Chinese medicine during pregnancy. Int. J. Clin. Exp. Med 8 (10), 19496–19500.

Chertok, I., 1999. Relief of breast engorgement for the Sabbath-observant Jewish woman. J. Obstet. Gynecol. Neonatal Nurs. 28 (4), 365–369.

Chou, C., 2017. Traditional postpartum practices and rituals: a qualitative systematic review (2007), by Cindy-Lee Dennis, Kenneth Fung, Sophie Grigoriadis, Gail Erlick Robinson, Sarah Romans and Lori Ross. The Embryo Project Encyclopedia. Available at: https://embryo.asu.edu/handle/10776/12977.

Choudhary, R., Gothwal, S., Nayan, S., Meena, B.S., 2017. Common ritualistic myths during pregnancy in Northern India. Int. J. Contemp. Pediatr. 4 (5), 1–4.

Choudhury, N., Moran, A.C., Alam, M.A., Ahsan, K.Z., Rashid, S.F., Streatfield, P.K., 2012. Beliefs and practices during pregnancy and childbirth in urban slums of Dhaka, Bangladesh. BMC Public Health 12 (1), 791.

Coffey, P.S., Brown, S.C., 2017. Umbilical cord-care practices in low- and middle-income countries: a systematic review. BMC Pregnancy Childbirth. 17, 68. https://doi.org/10.1186/s12884-017-1250-7.

Culhane-Pera, K.A., Sriphetcharawut, S., Thawsirichuchai, R., Yangyuenkun, W., Kunstadter, P., 2015. Afraid of delivering at the hospital or afraid of delivering at home: a qualitative study of Thai Hmong families' decision-making about maternity services. Matern. Child Health J. 19 (11), 2384–2392.

Curtis, E., Jones, R., Tipene-Leach, D., Walker, C., Loring, B., Paine, S.J., Reid, P., 2019. Why cultural safety rather than cultural competency is required to achieve health equity: a literature review and recommended definition. Int. J. Equity Health 18 (1), 174.

Darby, S.B., 2007. Pre- and perinatal care of hispanic families: implications for nurses. Nurs. Women's Health. 11 (2), 160–169.

Davis, D.L., Homer, C.S., 2016. Birthplace as the midwife's work place: how does place of birth impact on midwives? Women Birth 29 (5), 407–415.

Dean, R.A.K., 2010. Cultural competence: nursing in a multicultural society. Nurs. Women's Health. 14 (1), 50–59.

De Boer, H.J., Cotingting, C., 2014. Medicinal plants for women's healthcare in southeast Asia: a meta-analysis of their traditional use, chemical constituents, and pharmacology. J Ethnopharmacol. 151 (2), 747–767.

Dennis, C.L., Fung, K., Grigoriadis, S., Robinson, G.E., Romans, S., Ross, L., 2007. Traditional postpartum practices and rituals: a qualitative systematic review. Women's Health 3 (4), 487–502.

DeSouza, R., 2014. One woman's empowerment is another's oppression: Korean migrant mothers on giving birth in Aotearoa New Zealand. J. Transcult. Nurs. 25 (4), 348–356.

DeVito, J., 2019, April. Understanding the Orthodox Jewish family during childbirth. Nurs. Forum. 54 (2), 220–226.

Dike, P., 2013. Birth practices of Nigerian women: a literature review. African Journal of Midwifery and Women's Health. 7 (1), 39–48.

Du Gas, B.W., 1983. Introduction to Patient Care: A Comprehensive Approach to Nursing. WB Saunders Company, Philadelphia.

Durie, M., 2001, November. Cultural competence and medical practice in New Zealand Australian and New Zealand Boards and Council Conference (Vol. 22). School of Māori Studies, Massey University, Palmerston North.

El Hajj, M., Holst, L., 2020. Herbal medicine use during pregnancy: a review of the literature with a special focus on sub-Saharan Africa. Front Pharmacol. 9 (11), 866.

Esegbona-Adeigbe, S., 2011. Acquiring cultural competency in caring for black African women. Br. J. Midwifery. 19 (8), 489–496.

Esegbona-Adeigbe, S., 2018. Cultural qualities and antenatal care for black African women: a literature review. Br. J. Midwifery. 26 (8), 532–539.

Fantaye, A.W., Gunawardena, N., Yaya, S., 2019. Preferences for formal and traditional sources of childbirth and postnatal care among women in rural Africa: a systematic review. PloS one 14 (9), e0222110.

Fatmi, Z., Gulzar, A.Z., Kazi, A., 2005. Maternal and newborn care: practices and beliefs of traditional birth attendants in Sindh, Pakistan. East. Mediterr. Health J. 11 (2018-01-02), 226.

Frawley, J., Adams, J., Sibbritt, D., Steel, A., Broom, A., Gallois, C., 2013. Prevalence and determinants of complementary and alternative medicine use during pregnancy: results from a nationally representative sample of Australian pregnant women. Aust. N. Z. J. Obstet. Gynaecol. 53 (4), 347–352.

Gabrysch, S., Lema, C., Bedriñana, E., Bautista, M.A., Malca, R., Campbell, O.M., Miranda, J.J., 2009. Cultural adaptation of birthing services in rural Ayacucho, Peru. Bull. World Health Organ. 87, 724–729.

Gallegos, D., Vicca, N., Streiner, S., 2015. Breastfeeding beliefs and practices of African women living in Brisbane and Perth, Australia. Matern. Child Nutr. 11 (4), 727–736.

Gatrad, A.R., Ray, M., Sheikh, A., 2004. Hindu birth customs. Arch. Dis. Child. 89 (12), 1094–1097.

Gavelek, J.R., Kong, D.A., 2012. Learning: a process of enculturation. In: Seel, N.M. (Ed.), Encyclopedia of the Sciences of Learning. Springer, New York, pp. 2029–2032.

Ghosh, R., Sharma, A.K., 2010. Intra-and inter-household differences in antenatal care, delivery practices and postnatal care between last neonatal deaths and last surviving children in a peri-urban area of India. J. Biosoc. Sci. 42 (4), 511–530.

Giger, J.N., Davidhizar, R., 2002. The Giger and Davidhizar transcultural assessment model. J. Transcult. Nurs. 13 (3), 185–188.

Glei, D.A., Goldman, N., Rodrı-guez, G., 2003. Utilization of care during pregnancy in rural Guatemala: does obstetrical need matter? Soc Sci Med. 57 (12), 2447–2463.

Gul, S., Khalil, R., Yousafzai, M.T., Shoukat, F., 2014. Newborn care knowledge and practices among mothers attending pediatric outpatient clinic of a hospital in Karachi, Pakistan. Int. J. Health Sci. 8 (2), 167.

Hays, P.A., 2008. Addressing Cultural Complexities in Practice. American Psychological Association, Washington, DC.

Higginbottom, G.M., Safipour, J., Mumtaz, Z., Chiu, Y., Paton, P., Pillay, J., 2013. 'I have to do what I believe': Sudanese women's beliefs and resistance to hegemonic practices at home and during experiences of maternity care in Canada. BMC Pregnancy Childbirth 13 (1), 51.

Hill, N., Hunt, E., Hyrkäs, K., 2012. Somali immigrant women's health care experiences and beliefs regarding pregnancy and birth in the United States. J. Transcult. Nurs. 23 (1), 72–81.

Ingram, J., Johnson, D., Hamid, N., 2003. South Asian grandmothers' influence on breast feeding in Bristol. Midwifery. 19 (4), 318–327.

Ingram, J., Cann, K., Peacock, J., Potter, B., 2008. Exploring the barriers to exclusive breastfeeding in black and minority ethnic groups and young mothers in the UK. Matern. Child Nutr. 4 (3), 171–180. https://doi.org/10.1111/j.1740-8709.2007.00129.x.

John, L.J., Shantakumari, N., 2015. Herbal medicines use during pregnancy: a review from the middle East. Oman Med. J. 30 (4), 229–236. https://doi.org/10.5001/omj.2015.4.

Jordal, M., Wahlberg, A., 2018. Challenges in providing quality care for women with female genital cutting in Sweden–a literature review. Sex. Reprod. Healthc. 17, 91–96.

Joseph, F.I., Earland, J., 2019. A qualitative exploration of the sociocultural determinants of exclusive breastfeeding practices among rural mothers. North West Nigeria. Int. Breastfeed. J. 14 (1), 1–11.

Kang, H.K., 2014. Influence of culture and community perceptions on birth and perinatal care of immigrant women: doulas' perspective. J. Perinat. Educ. 23 (1), 25.

Kanu, I.A., 2019. An Igwebuike approach to the study of African traditional naming ceremony and baptism. J. Reli. Human Relat. 11 (1), 25–52.

Kaphle, S., Hancock, H., Newman, L.A., 2013. Childbirth traditions and cultural perceptions of safety in Nepal: critical spaces to ensure the survival of mothers and newborns in remote mountain villages. Midwifery 29 (10), 1173–1181.

Kaplan, RA., 2004. The rules of halacha. Available at: https://www.aish.com/jl/m/pm/48932007.html.

Kim-Godwin, Y.S., 2003. Postpartum beliefs and practices among non-Western cultures. MCN Am. J. Matern. Child Nurs. 28 (2), 74–78.

Kirshner, D., Meng, L., 2012. Enculturation and acculturation. In: Seel, N.M. (Ed.), Encyclopedia of the Sciences of Learning. Springer, New York.

Kridli, S.A.O., Ilori, O.M., Verriest, H.L., 2013. Health beliefs and practices related to pregnancy and childcare in Qatar: a qualitative study. J. Nurs. Educ. Prac. 3 (2), 1.

Lau, Y., 2012. Traditional Chinese pregnancy restrictions, health-related quality of life and perceived stress among pregnant women in Macao, China. Asian Nurs. Res. 6 (1), 27–34.

Lauderdale, J., 2008. Transcultural perspectives in childbearing. In: Andrews, M.M., Boyle, J.S. (Eds.), Transcultural Concepts in Nursing Care, 5th ed. Lippincott, Williams & Wilkins, Philadelphia, pp. 85–115.

Manley, K., Sanders, K., Cardiff, S., Webster, J., 2011. Effective workplace culture: the attributes, enabling factors and consequences of a new concept. Int. Prac. Develop. J. 1 (2), 1–29.

Mannion, R., Davies, H., 2018. Understanding organisational culture for healthcare quality improvement. BMJ, 363.

Major, M., 2020. What postpartum care looks like around the world, and why the U.S. is missing the mark. https://www.healthline.com/health/pregnancy/what-post-childbirth-care-looks-like-around-the-world-and-why-the-u-s-is-missing-the-mark.

Markey, K., Tilki, M., Taylor, G., 2018. Understanding nurses' concerns when caring for patients from diverse cultural and ethnic backgrounds. J. Clin. Nurs. 27 (12), e259–e268.

Martínez Pérez, G., Pascual García, A., 2013. Nutritional taboos among the Fullas in Upper River region, the Gambia. J. Anthropology 2013, 1–9.

McKenzie, K., Tuck, A., Noh, M.S., 2011. Moving traditional Caribbean medicine practices into healthcare in Canada. Ethn. Inequal. Health Soc. Care 4 (2), 60–70.

Memon, J., Holakouie-Naieni, K., Majdzadeh, R., Yekaninejad, M.S., Garmaroudi, G., Raza, O., Nematollahi, S., 2019. Knowledge, attitude, and practice among mothers about newborn care in Sindh, Pakistan. BMC Pregnancy Childbirth 19 (1), 1–9.

Mirzabagi, E., Deepak, N.N., Koski, A., Tripathi, V., 2013. Uterotonic use during childbirth in Uttar Pradesh: accounts from community members and health providers. Midwifery 29 (8), 902–910.

Moore, K., 2007. Naming traditions from around the world. https://www.ethnictechnologies.com/blog/2018/10/2/naming-traditions-from-around-the-world.

Morrison, J., Thapa, R., Basnet, M., Budhathoki, B., Tumbahangphe, K., Manandhar, D., et al., 2014. Exploring the first delay: a qualitative study of home deliveries in Makwanpur district Nepal. BMC Pregnancy Childbirth 14 (1), 1–7.

Moses, B.E., Emma, E.J., Christopher, C.M., Enobong, I.B., Theresa, B.E., 2012. Effect of calabash chalk on the histomorphology of the gastro-oesophageal tract of growing wistar rats. Malay. J. Med. Sci. 19 (1), 30–35.

Mukhopadhyay, S., Sarkar, A., 2009. Pregnancy-related food habits among women of rural Sikkim, India. Public Health Nutr. 12 (12), 2317–2322.

Murray, L., Windsor, C., Parker, E., Tewfik, O., 2010. The experiences of African women giving birth in Brisbane, Australia. Health Care Women Int. 31 (5), 458–472.

Naser, E., Mackey, S., Arthur, D., Klainin-Yobas, P., Chen, H., Creedy, D.K., 2012. An exploratory study of traditional birthing practices of Chinese, Malay and Indian women in Singapore. Midwifery. 28 (6), e865–e871.

Noble, A., Rom, M., Newsome-Wicks, M., Engelhardt, K., Woloski-Wruble, A., 2009. Jewish laws, customs, and practice in labor, delivery, and postpartum care. J. Transcult. Nurs. 20 (3), 323–333.

NMC, 2018. Code of Professional Conduct: Professional Standards for Nurses and Midwives Nursing & Midwifery Council, London.

Obuna, J.A., Umeora, O.U.J., 2014. Perception of labor pain and utilization of obstetric analgesia by Igbo women of Southeast Nigeria. J. Obstet. Anaesth. Crit. Care. 4 (1), 18.

Ocho, O.N., Moorley, C., Lootawan, K.A., 2018. Fathers' presence in the birth room–implications for professional practice in the Caribbean. Contemp. Nurse. 54 (6), 617–629.

O'Connell, R., Downe, S., 2009. A metasynthesis of midwives' experience of hospital practice in publicly funded settings: compliance, resistance and authenticity. Health. 13 (6), 589–609.

Ozioma, E.O.J., Chinwe, O.A.N., 2019. Herbal medicines in African traditional medicine. Herb. Med 10, 191–214.

Parisa, B., Reza, N., Afsaneh, R., Sarieh, P., 2016. Cultural safety. Holistic nursing practice. 30 (1), 33–38.

Paul, M., Iyioriobhe, E., 2017. Public health of birth and loss: rituals from around the world. Available at: https://unthsc-ir.tdl.org/handle/20.500.12503/27668.

Phiri, J., Dietsch, E., Bonner, A., 2010. Cultural safety and its importance for Australian midwifery practice. Collegian 17 (3), 105–111.

Posmontier, B., Horowitz, J.A., 2004. Postpartum practices and depression prevalences: technocentric and ethnokinship cultural perspectives. J. Transcult. Nurs. 15 (1), 34–43.

Posmontier, B., Horowitz, J.A., 2007. Postpartum practices and depression prevalences: technocentric and ethnokinship cultural perspectives. J. Transcult. Nurs. http://.tcn.sagepub.com/cgi/content.

Raman, S., Srinivasan, K., Kurpad, A., Razee, H., Ritchie, J., 2014. 'Nothing special, everything is Maamuli': socio-cultural and family practices influencing the perinatal period in urban India. PloS one 9 (11), e111900.

Raman, S., Nicholls, R., Ritchie, J., Razee, H., Shafiee, S., 2016. How natural is the supernatural? Synthesis of the qualitative literature from low and middle income countries on cultural practices and traditional beliefs influencing the perinatal period. Midwifery 39, 87–97.

Rassool, G.H. (Ed.), 2014. Cultural competence in caring for muslim patients. Basingstoke: Macmillan International Higher Education.

Rice, P.L., Naksook, C., Watson, L., 1999. The experiences of postpartum hospital stay and returning home among Thai mothers in Australia. Midwifery 15 (1), 47–57.

Roya, A., 2017. Necessity of Samskaras in Modern Society. Int. J. Innovat. Res. Advan. Study 4 (6), 79–83.

Rytterström, P., Cedersund, E., Arman, M., 2009. Care and caring culture as experienced by nurses working in different care environments: a phenomenological–hermeneutic study. Int. J. Nurs. Stud. 46 (5), 689–698.

Sacks, E., Moss, W.J., Winch, P.J., Thuma, P., van Dijk, J.H., Mullany, L.C., 2015. Skin, thermal and umbilical cord care practices for neonates in southern, rural Zambia: a qualitative study. BMC Pregnancy Childbirth 15 (1), 1–11.

Schein, E.H., 2010. Organizational Culture and Leadership, vol. 2. John Wiley & Sons, San Francisco.

Sefiha, O., 2007. Ethnocentrism. Black. Encyclo. Sociol, 1–2.

Semenic, S.E., Callister, L.C., Feldman, P., 2004. Giving birth: the voices of Orthodox Jewish women living in Canada. J. Obstet. Gynecol. Neonatal Nurs. 33 (1), 80–87.

Semrau, K.E., Herlihy, J., Grogan, C., Musokotwane, K., Yeboah-Antwi, K., Mbewe, R., et al., 2016. Effectiveness of 4% chlorhexidine umbilical cord care on neonatal mortality in Southern Province, Zambia (ZamCAT): a cluster-randomised controlled trial. Lancet Glob. Health 4 (11), e827–e836.

Shewamene, Z., Tinashe, D., Caroline, A.S., 2017. The use of traditional medicine in maternity care among African women in Africa and the diaspora: a systematic review. BMC Complement. Altern. Med. 17 (1) 1–1.

Sperstad, R.A., Werner, J.S., 2005. Coming to the cultural in-between: nursing insights from a Hmong birth case study. J. Obstet. Gynecol. Neonatal Nurs. 34 (6), 682–688.

Steinman, L., Doescher, M., Keppel, G.A., Pak-Gorstein, S., Graham, E., Haq, A., et al., 2010. Understanding infant feeding beliefs, practices and preferred nutrition education and health provider approaches: an exploratory study with Somali mothers in the USA. Matern. Child Nutr. 6 (1), 67–88.

Syed, U., Khadka, N., Khan, A., Wall, S., 2008. Care-seeking practices in South Asia: using formative research to design program interventions to save newborn lives. J. Perinat. 28 (2), S9–S13.

Szczepura, A., 2005. Access to health care for ethnic minority populations. Postgrad. Med. J 81 (953), 141–147.

Tewari, P.V., 1997. Introduction to Kashyap Samhita. Chaukhambha Vishwabharati, Varanasi.

Textor, L., Tiedje, K., Yawn, B., 2013. Mexican and Somali immigrant breastfeeding initiation and counseling: a qualitative study of practices. Minn. Med. 96 (12), 46–50.

Tortello, R., 2021. A Time to Live Jamaican Birth Rituals. https://old.jamaica-gleaner.com/pages/history/story0079.html

Tory, D., 2013. Postpartum Culture, The Jewish naming ceremony. https://welcomebabycare.com/postpartum-culture-jewish-naming-ceremony/.

Ugwa, E.A., 2016. Nutritional practices and taboos among pregnant women attending antenatal care at general hospital in Kano, Northwest Nigeria. Ann. Med. Health Sci. Res. 6 (2), 109–114.

Vallely, L.M., Homiehombo, P., Kelly, A.M., Vallely, A., Homer, C.S., Whittaker, A., 2013. Exploring women's perspectives of access to care during pregnancy and childbirth: a qualitative study from rural Papua New Guinea. Midwifery. 29 (10), 1222–1229.

Van Andel, T., de Boer, H.J., Barnes, J., Vandebroek, I., 2014. Medicinal plants used for menstrual disorders in Latin America, the Caribbean, sub-Saharan Africa, South and Southeast Asia and their uterine properties: a review. J. Ethnopharmacol. 155 (2), 992–1000.

Vasilevski, V., Carolan-Olah, M., 2016. Food taboos and nutrition-related pregnancy concerns among Ethiopian women. J. Clin. Nurs. 25 (19–20), 3069–3075.

Volpato, G., Godinez, D., 2006. Medicinal foods in Cuba: promoting health in the household. In: Pieroni, A., Price, L.L. (Eds.), Eating and Healing: Traditional Food as Medicine. Haworth Press, Binghamton, NY, pp. 213–235.

Wagner, C., Mannion, R., Hammer, A., Groene, O., Arah, O.A., Dersarkissian, M., Suñol, R., DUQuE Project Consortium, 2014. The associations between organizational culture, organizational structure and quality management in European hospitals. Int. J. Qual. Health Care. 26 (Suppl 1), 74–80.

Weber, S.E., 1996. Cultural aspects of pain in childbearing women. J. Obstet. Gynecol. Neonatal Nurs. 25 (1), 67–72.

Wehbe-Alamah, H., Hammonds, L.S., Stanley, D., 2021. Culturally congruent care from the perspectives of Judaism, Christianity, and Islam. J. Transcult. Nurs. 32 (2), 119–128.

Weiss, H., Polonsky, J., Bailey, R., Hankins, C., Halperin, D., Schmid, G., 2007. Male Circumcision. Global Trends and Determinants of Prevalence, Safety and Acceptability. World Health Organization, Joint United Nations Programme on HIV/AIDS, Geneva, Switzerland.

WHO, 2007. Male circumcision: global trends and determinants of prevalence, safety and acceptability. https://www.who.int/reproductivehealth/publications/rtis/9789241596169/en/.

WHO, 2013. WHO recommendations on postnatal care of the mother and newborn. World Health Organization. Available at: https://apps.who.int/iris/bitstream/handle/10665/97603/9789241506649_eng.pdf?sequence=1&isAllowed=y.

WHO, 2017. Culture matters: using a cultural contexts of health approach to enhance policy-making. Available at: https://www.euro.who.int/-data/assets/pdf_file/0009/334269/14780_World-Health-Organisation_Context-of-Health_TEXT-AW-WEB.pdf.

Wilcken, A., Keil, T., Dick, B., 2010. Traditional male circumcision in eastern and southern Africa: a systematic review of prevalence and complications. Bull. World Health Organ. 88, 907–914.

Withers, M., Kharazmi, N., Lim, E., 2018. Traditional beliefs and practices in pregnancy, childbirth and postpartum: A review of the evidence from Asian countries. Midwifery. 56, 158–170.

Worthman, C.M., Plotsky, P.M., Schechter, D.S., Cummings, C.A. (Eds.), 2010. Formative Experiences: the Interaction of Caregiving, Culture, and Developmental Psychobiology. Cambridge University Press, Cambridge.

Xie, A., Huang, H., Kong, F., 2020. Relationship between food composition and its cold/hot properties: a statistical study. J. Agric. Food Res, 100043.

Xu, T., Yue, Q., Wang, Y., Murray, J., Sobel, H., 2018. Childbirth and early newborn care practices in 4 provinces in China: a comparison with WHO recommendations. Glob. Health Sci. Pract. 6 (3), 565–573.

Yavuz, A.Y., Derya, Y.A., Hacer, G.Ö.K., 2020. Traditional practices in infant care in Eastern Region of Turkey. Mid. Black Sea J. Health Sci. 6 (2), 257–266.

Young, S.M., Benyshek, D.C., 2010. In search of human placentophagy: a cross-cultural survey of human placenta consumption, disposal practices, and cultural beliefs. Ecol. Food Nutr. 49 (6), 467–484.

Zhou, Q., Younger, K.M., Kearney, J.M., 2010. An exploration of the knowledge and attitudes towards breast-feeding among a sample of Chinese mothers in Ireland. BMC Public Health. 10 (1), 722.

Barriers to Transcultural Care

INTRODUCTION

Caring for women from different cultures can lead to barriers to effective care. These barriers are not insurmountable and should be recognised and solutions found. In this chapter, you will explore the barriers that may commonly arise during midwifery practice. An examination of the multidimensional viewpoint of the woman when facing these barriers and how this can be addressed within the parameters of safe midwifery practice will be provided.

Individual Barriers

REDUCED KNOWLEDGE OF MATERNITY SERVICES

Women's lack of knowledge of how the healthcare service works within the UK has been known to create barriers to accessing maternity care. The main issues include lack of recognition of importance of antenatal care by migrant women in their new home country, lack of familiarity with multiple health providers and not knowing what to expect during childbirth (Hill et al., 2012; Higginbottom et al., 2019; Hoban and Liamputtong, 2013). The lack of understanding of the role of healthcare professionals has also been noted as a barrier to accessing care; Feldman (2013) reported that this was often a factor in nonattendance due to mistrust. For many mothers, maternity services represent a complex system that they do not understand (McLeish and Redshaw, 2019).

Women new to the UK may have different expectations of pregnancy care due to how maternity services are usually provided in their own countries. Differences in how to access services can delay the utilisation of maternity care. In other countries, access may be made directly to a doctor where provisions are made for pregnancy care. The need to attend a hospital or a community centre may be unusual for a migrant woman. There may be no recommended time of reporting pregnancy in the woman's country of origin with reliance on the culturally accepted time that pregnancy should be revealed.

Having to navigate the healthcare system when there are language barriers poses difficulties for women. In addition, even if there is no language barrier, advice on how to access pregnancy care is not advertised in a way that appeals to all women. Family or friends usually provide information about accessing pregnancy care to some women hence, incorrect or inappropriate information may be given. Unfortunately, the information on how maternity units can be accessed and how they operate is not readily available to all women. Advocacy groups, in particular, have commented on barriers created by the concept of 'open door' access in the UK which assumed that because everybody was welcome, services were accessible and there was no need to promote services in different languages or formats or target minority ethnic communities proactively (Cha, 2013). All these factors are underlying problems, which may influence women approaching services for healthcare or advice. If access is made, other issues arise, ranging from language/communication barriers to culturally insensitive services.

Exercise

Please review the following scenario regarding access to maternity services.

Tunde is a Nigerian woman who has recently arrived in the UK and is currently 10 weeks pregnant. She is unaware that she needs to register with a GP and decides that she will go to a hospital if she has any concerns about her pregnancy. Her main priority is to get used to living in the UK.

Learning Activity

1. What do you think are the main issues here and how could they have been addressed?

Practice Point

Understanding why women are not aware of maternity services is important. It is not always clear to midwives what the issues may be, and it is obvious that women are unclear too. Community engagement is essential for addressing this issue as often midwives are only aware that a woman is pregnant once she presents for pregnancy care. The presence of midwives in community centres and GP surgeries is usual as they often conduct antenatal and postnatal clinics in these settings. Liaison within these settings could facilitate community engagement by advertising midwives and maternity services.

REDUCED ENGAGEMENT WITH MATERNITY SERVICES

There are several reasons why women may find it difficult to engage with maternity services once access is made. A major issue is the lack of respect women have experienced or heard from family and friends. A deep underlying fear and distrust of services linked to trauma and negative experiences of services make engaging with maternity care difficult for some women. McLeish and Redshaw (2019) reported that mothers reported negative experiences of interactions with staff and felt processed through a system by professionals who followed procedures without really noticing the woman in front of them so that mothers were made to feel like they were just part of the system. The impact of this on the cultural identity of the woman cannot be overlooked.

The absence of respect and dignity in maternity care creates stress, anxiety and fear of communicating cultural views. Women with lower socioeconomic status are more likely to report that they were not treated respectfully, were not spoken to in a way they could understand during their maternity care and were not heard when they expressed concerns (Lindquist et al., 2015). Unfortunately, women from culturally diverse backgrounds may also be less likely to not have their cultural views or wishes respected. This leads to dissatisfaction with the care provision and reduced engagement.

Consequently, negative experiences of healthcare lead to women expecting poor treatment. This is particularly prevalent among women with a first language other than English, who felt that the language barrier made them vulnerable to prejudice and discrimination (Maternity Action, 2018). Therefore, the midwife must focus on ensuring that once women access maternity care, provision is made to address any concerns or wishes that they may have. The booking interview is an opportunity to ensure that the woman fully accepts the pregnancy care plan, and she understands the importance. Moreover, ensuring the care plan is delivered in a culturally acceptable way and does not create cultural barriers is crucial. The significance of this stance not being taken leads to women becoming disillusioned and unable to continue to engage with maternity services.

Exercise

Review the following scenario highlighting the impact of disrespect during pregnancy care.

Johanna is 29 weeks pregnant and has already been booked for pregnancy. However, at the booking appointment and the follow-up appointment, she felt her views about her pregnancy were not listened to by the midwife. At times she felt the midwife talked down to her and made derogatory remarks about her culture. This experience and views she has heard from friends have reduced her confidence in discussing her wishes for her pregnancy with the midwife.

Learning Activity

1. What do you think will be the potential impact of this experience on Johanna's pregnancy?
2. Do you think that this may be a common occurrence in your workplace?
3. Think about how you would feel if you were disrespected in any situation as a service user or customer.

In 2011, the White Ribbon Alliance produced the Respectful Maternity Care Charter: The Universal Rights of Childbearing Women (Copeland, 2019). The lead up to this was the prevalence of reports of violations of women's rights in childbirth from the human rights community. The World Health Organization (WHO) released a statement in 2014 reasserting the fundamental human rights of women in childbirth (WHO, 2014). Hence, there has been a focus on addressing disrespect and abuse as the reasons there are systemic failures to uphold human rights standards.

McConville (2014) discusses the key elements of respectful maternity care, and the rights women are entitled to (Box. 5.1). Lack of these rights is likely to decrease women's engagement with maternity services.

Maternity services have recognised these rights in the UK and taken steps to improve women's perception of maternity services (see Case 5.1).

BOX 5.1 ■ Respectful Maternity Care Charter: Universal Rights of Women and Newborn

1. Everyone has the right to freedom from harm and ill-treatment.
   No one is allowed to physically hurt you or your newborn. You should both be taken care of gently and compassionately and receive assistance when experiencing pain or discomfort.
2. Everyone has the right to information, informed consent and respect for their choices and preferences, including companion of choice during maternity care and refusal of medical procedures.
   No one is allowed to force you or do things to you or your newborn without your knowledge or consent. Every woman has the right to autonomy, to receive information and provide informed consent or refusal for care. Every parent or guardian has the right to receive information and provide informed consent or refusal for their newborn's care, in the newborn's best interests, unless otherwise provided by law.
3. Everyone has the right to privacy and confidentiality.
   No one is allowed to share your or your newborn's personal or medical information, including all records and images, without your consent. Yours' and your newborn's privacy must be protected, except as necessary for healthcare providers to convey information for continuity of care.
4. Everyone is their own person from the moment of birth and has the right to be treated with dignity and respect.
   No one is allowed to humiliate, verbally abuse, speak about or touch you or your newborn in a degrading or disrespectful manner. You and your newborn baby must be cared for with respect and compassion.
5. Everyone has the right to equality, freedom from discrimination and equitable care.
   No one is allowed to discriminate against you or your newborn because of something they think or do not like about either one of you. Equality requires that pregnant women have the same protections under the law as they would when they are not pregnant, including the right to make decisions about what happens to their bodies.
6. Everyone has the right to healthcare and the highest attainable level of health.
   No one may prevent you or your newborn from getting the healthcare needed or deny or withhold care from either one of you. You and your newborn are entitled to the highest quality care, provided on time, in a clean and safe environment, by providers trained in current best practices.
7. Everyone has the right to liberty, autonomy, self-determination and freedom from arbitrary detention.
   No one is allowed to detain you or your newborn in a healthcare facility, even if you cannot pay for services received.
8. Every child has the right to be with their parents or guardians.
   No one is allowed to separate you from your newborn without your consent. You and your newborn have the right to remain together at all times, even if your newborn is born small, premature or with medical conditions that require extra care.
9. Every child has the right to an identity and nationality from birth.
   No one is allowed to deny your newborn birth registration, even if they die shortly after birth, or deny the nationality, your newborn is legally entitled to.
10. Everyone has the right to adequate nutrition and clean water.
    No one is allowed to prevent you and your newborn from having adequate nutrition, clean water or a healthy environment. You have the right to information and support on child nutrition and the advantages of breastfeeding.

Reproduced with permission from White Ribbon Alliance, 2018. White Ribbon Alliance. Available at: https://www.whiteribbonalliance.org/respectful-maternity-care-charter/.

Break the Silence is a White Ribbon Alliance programme highlighting disrespect and abuse in maternity services and women's rights to be treated well during childbirth. The impact of disrespectful maternity care leads to severe health disparities for pregnant women, particularly women from ethnic minority backgrounds. The following case study highlights how this can be addressed.

CASE 5.1 TACKLING DISRESPECTFUL CARE IN A LONDON MATERNITY UNIT (COPELAND, 2019)

In 2010, a National Health Service (NHS) teaching hospital was subject to an investigation by the Care Quality Commission on attitudes to women's care following the deaths of five pregnant women within 2 years.

Midwifery leaders responded with a range of initiatives, one of which was to provide staff with training in Respectful Care, using White Ribbon Alliance's RMC Charter, graphic film and a role play specially devised by midwives. According to the Director of Midwifery and Divisional Nurse Director who instituted the training in respectful care for maternity staff, satisfaction levels amongst women attending maternity care improved dramatically:

'Women were petrified to come to the hospital, because of all they had heard and read in the media', so when a White Ribbon Alliance member in the UK showed the Director of Midwifery the short film about Respectful Maternity Care, 'Break the Silence', she said 'how wonderful, we need to be doing this here. I made this mandatory training for staff. With our ethnic mix, we made it clear that what might be right in some cultures is not okay at work. We work as a team here, not as a hierarchy. Some staff have learned to leave their culture at home and to be professional at work'.

It is essential to recognise from this case study the impact of recognising women's needs and how important it is for health professionals to facilitate the cultural context of the woman and not their own.

LANGUAGE AND LITERACY BARRIERS

Problems with written and verbal communication relating largely to language barriers are common challenges for pregnant women. Lack of interpreters has led to negative healthcare experiences and difficulties in accessing health services (Knight et al., 2019). Without interpretation, even the basic cultural needs of the woman are unachievable. Women become frustrated when they cannot communicate effectively with the midwife and do not see the point of attending pregnancy care. Even in the presence of interpretation services, other frustrations arise as communication between healthcare professionals and women could be inefficient, especially if the expectations of a consultation differ.

Some women are at a particular disadvantage due to lower levels of literacy and English language skills and are also inhibited by cultural factors, such as the use of male interpreters in maternity or sexual health services or when disclosing experiences of domestic or sexual violence (Nellums et al., 2018). Sometimes too many professionals are included in a consultation, or too much information is given at once, which overwhelms the woman. Maternity care counselling on health education and promotion can risk bombarding the woman with a wall of information that does not apply to individual needs and concerns (Origlia Ikhilor et al., 2019).

Lack of effective communication can also lead to misunderstandings between the woman and midwife, resulting in the woman's dissatisfaction with her maternity care (Murray et al., 2010; Higginbottom et al., 2015; Wojnar, 2015). Women begin to disengage with services when they feel their views are not being heard or their culture respected. In some cases, it has meant that women did not comply with midwifery advice and recommendations (Murray et al., 2010; Higginbottom et al., 2015). Decision making is important to pregnant women, and language barriers lead to a lack of control at an extremely important period (Murray et al., 2010; Wojnar, 2015). Women who face this lack of control experience anxiety and dismay at not knowing how their pregnancy care should be conducted (Murray et al., 2010).

Low health literacy, cultural barriers and limited English proficiency have been coined the 'triple threat' to effective health communication by The Joint Commission (Schyve, 2007; Hughson et al., 2018). Literacy in the home language is a barrier for certain groups such as Bengalis and Somalis; the absence of a written language or reliance on an oral rather than a literary tradition limits the ability to convey information (Cha, 2013). Pregnancy information in translated languages may not be useful to some women. Also, women, whilst having some skills in reading and writing, may have a cultural tradition of folk medicine, for which information is typically conveyed orally, creating a disadvantage when patients adopt the stance of reading and writing in Western healthcare systems (Singleton and Krause, 2009). Reading and writing skills vary for women from other cultures because language structures and educational opportunities vary from country to country (Singleton and Krause, 2009). In addition, a significant difference could be a different alphabet system or cultural differences in pictorial health information. Hence, although some women may learn to speak English as a second language, reading English may be more difficult.

HEALTH LITERACY

The ability to understand health-related information can also create barriers to accessing and engaging with maternity services. Low health literacy can adversely affect a woman's ability to navigate the healthcare system whilst pregnant (Shieh et al., 2009). A woman is considered to be health literate if she knows how to access, understand, appraise and apply health-related information within healthcare (Sørensen et al., 2012). In addition, health literacy requires motivation to navigate a healthcare system. Consequently, health literate women are able to negotiate, question and demand healthcare that meets their individual needs. The presence of a language or literacy barrier instantly makes this unrealistic. This puts women at a disadvantage as their wishes and needs during pregnancy may not be heard. In mothers, paying attention to health literacy status is important for two reasons: first, pregnancy may be a woman's first exposure to the healthcare system; therefore, working on this complex system for the first time can be complicated, even with sufficient literacy skills (Asadi et al., 2020). Even women with high literacy may experience problems learning new information and following guidelines. The second disadvantage is that a woman's health status and her understanding of health information directly affects her baby before pregnancy, during pregnancy and into childhood (Asadi et al., 2020).

A matrix adapted from Sørensen et al. (2012) (Table 5.1) identifies how health literacy can impact a pregnant woman.

Practice Point

Good communication between healthcare professionals and women is essential. It should be supported by evidence-based written information tailored to the woman's needs. Treatment and care, and the information women are given about it, should be culturally appropriate. Such care should also be accessible to women with additional needs such as physical, sensory or learning disabilities and to women who are unable speak or read English (National Institute for Health and Care Excellence, 2016).

STIGMA

Stigma is the linking of undesirable characteristics to individuals who are in some way identified as different to others. Often stigma refers to attitudes and emotional reactions, whereas

TABLE 5.1 ■ Matrix with Four Competencies of Health Literacy Applied to Three Health Domains

	Access/Obtain Information Relevant to Health	Understand Information Relevant to Health	Process/Appraise Information Relevant to Health	Apply/Use Information Relevant to Health
Healthcare	Ability to access information on medical or clinical issues	Ability to understand medical information and derive meaning	Ability to interpret and evaluate medical information	Ability to make informed decisions on medical issues
Disease prevention	Ability to access information on risk factors for health	Ability to understand information on risk factors and derive meaning	Ability to interpret and evaluate information on risk factors for health	Ability to make informed decisions on risk factors for health
Health promotion	Ability to update oneself on determinants of health in the social and physical environment	Ability to understand information on determinants of health in the social and physical environment and derive meaning	Ability to interpret and evaluate information on health determinants in the social and physical environment	Ability to make informed decisions on health determinants in the social and physical environment

Modified from Sørensen, K., Van den Broucke, S., Fullam, J., Doyle, G., Pelikan, J., Slonska, Z., Brand, H., 2012. Health literacy and public health: a systematic review and integration of definitions and models. *BMC Public Health*. 12 (1), 1–13.

discrimination refers to the behavioural enactment of stigma. Stigma can present in different forms (Table 5.2).

It is believed that cultural beliefs influence stigma, hence the impact on women's health-seeking behaviour for particular illnesses (Fig. 5.1). The dominant cultural stigma beliefs of a country affect the behaviour of its citizens, independent of their own beliefs, supporting the idea that stigma is a cultural phenomenon (Phelan et al., 2014). It is stated that the power of stigma emerges within a cultural system as beliefs about what is or what ought to be – that are shared by the members of a social system and transmitted to new members' (Link and Phelan, 2001). The

TABLE 5.2 ■ Behavioural Enactment of Stigma

Public stigma	Negative attitudes within society or direct discrimination directed towards individuals with a mental health condition
Structural stigma	When the policies and actions of private and government institutions restrict the opportunities of people with mental illness (intentional or unintentional)
Self-stigma	The internalising of negative views of society results in self-limiting behaviour, e.g. I won't apply for a job as I can't do it because I'm useless (with depression) etc
Stigma by association	Experience of stigma by those connected to an individual with a mental health condition, e.g. a family member or friend

Reproduced with permission from Mental Health Foundation, 2021. Stigma and discrimination. https://www.mentalhealth.org.uk/a-to-z/s/stigma-and-discrimination.

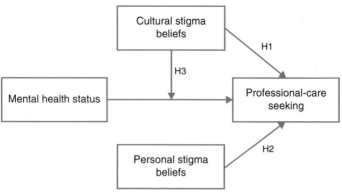

Fig. 5.1   Impact of stigma on health-seeking behaviour. (Reproduced with permission from Bracke et al, 2019.)

consideration of stigma as a cultural phenomenon that differs across countries has several conceptual implications. One is that it implies that citizens of the same country or members of the same culture share stigmatising perceptions and attitudes, at least to some extent (Bracke et al., 2019). For example, culture is said to determine how much stigma immigrant women attach to mental illness (O'Mahony and Donnelly, 2007).

Stigma about mental illness may keep women from ethnic minority groups from seeking treatment for common mental disorders (Das et al., 2006) and might be an important factor in explaining disparities in care. It is believed that individuals of countries with a strongly stigmatising culture are less likely to utilise professional mental healthcare services, regardless of their personal stigma beliefs (Bracke et al., 2019).

Impact of cultural stigma on health-seeking behaviour research with recently arrived African migrant women in London highlighted a stigma surrounding postnatal depression in their country of origin and the UK (Babatunde and Moreno-Leguizamon, 2012). The risk of being stigmatised prevents women from disclosing their concerns to midwives, creating a cultural barrier to appropriate treatment and care. In some migrant communities, attitude to mental illness is derogatory, with women fearing that if their mental health problems become public knowledge, they would be exposed and stigmatised by families and communities (Wheeler, 1998; Gilbert et al., 2004).

Therefore, cultural and social attitudes and stigma associated with certain medical conditions, can affect women's decisions to seek treatment. In particular, people with mental health needs or who experience trauma or torture may mistrust health professionals. Previous poor services experiences, including potentially discriminatory or abusive situations, add to this lack of trust (Nellums et al., 2018).

Practice Point

Often stigma is not easily identifiable as being the barrier to women accessing care. Communicating with a woman on any health conditions that she may have that are culturally unacceptable can be difficult. Therefore, your understanding of the impact of cultural stigma on a woman's health-seeking behaviour in pregnancy is crucial.

RECENT MIGRANTS

Gaps in service provision that impact the integration and service utilisation of migrant families is an issue; studies in diverse populations show that health services struggle to understand and meet migrant women's needs (Phillimore, 2015). Resettlement in a new country can result in differential access to care due to social disadvantages (Bradby et al., 2015; Keygnaert et al., 2016). Other barriers to accessing optimal maternity care for migrant women include low socioeconomic status and social disadvantage, which contribute to differential access to health and maternity care (Pangas et al., 2019).

The common barriers to healthcare for migrant women include language literacy, access issues and the provision of culturally inappropriate care and experiences of discrimination and racism (All Party Parliamentary Group on Refugees, 2017). Living between two cultures has a profound impact on women who are trying to maintain culturally significant constructs of mothering while simultaneously striving to provide the best for their children (Pangas et al., 2019). Women may be regularly offered care that contrasts with their culturally embedded notions of motherhood or does not accommodate their cultural beliefs (Niner et al., 2013; Russo et al., 2015; Stewart et al., 2015).

Most women will tend to adopt the recommended maternal practices of their host country (Carolan and Cassar, 2010; Hill et al., 2012; Owens et al., 2016). This stance may be due to pressures or the need to acculturate, or women may welcome this chance to submerge themselves in a culture and a new way of doing things. However, often women are required to compromise, re-evaluate or assimilate their beliefs (Carolan and Cassar, 2010; Lillrank, 2015; Russo et al., 2015; Wojnar, 2015). If this is the case, satisfaction and engagement with maternity services are impacted. Women may feel marginalised by services that are focused on efficiency leading to inadequate resourcing and information, leaving women vulnerable to misunderstanding, particularly if they had low literacy levels or lacked the language proficiency to negotiate care (Murray et al., 2010; Shafiei et al., 2012; Stapleton et al., 2013).

REFUGEES AND ASYLUM SEEKERS

Pregnant asylum seekers experience significant barriers to accessing maternity services in the UK. A review found that these barriers often relate to language differences and practical challenges associated with their status. The provision of interpreter services and training for healthcare professionals could improve maternity support for these women.

Many women arrive in the country having received no maternity care and experience difficulties accessing appropriate services once in the UK (Knight et al., 2019).

The needs of refugees and asylum seekers are unique; hence, they face additional pressures that impact their cultural identity. The terms asylum seeker and refugee are used interchangeably. The terms by Asif et al. (2015) (Table 5.3) provide clarification of women who are asylum seekers or refugees and their legal status.

Pregnant asylum seekers also face challenges related to barriers to accessing care due to language issues and knowledge of maternity service (McKnight et al., 2019). In addition, the consequence of immigration law impacts women's access to maternity services (Higginbottom et al., 2019). Fear and anxiety may also influence women's health-seeking behaviour, whether due to unfamiliarity of the system or fear of prosecution if awaiting asylum (Ndirangu and Evans, 2009).

This fear and anxiety have also been attributed to cultural insensitivity (Higginbottom et al., 2019). Recent evidence suggests that asylum seekers often have negative experiences with midwives mirroring negative public opinions, demonstrating poor attitudes, rudeness and racism (McLeish and Alliance, 2002; Briscoe and Lavender, 2009). There is evidence that women both

TABLE 5.3 ■ **Legal Status and Asylum Seekers**

Immigration Status	Definition	Legal Status
Asylum seeker	A woman who flees from perceived risk enters a host country and informs the authorities that she wishes to claim asylum	The woman can remain in the country while awaiting the outcome of her claim She has no legal rights to work, study or claim benefits in the UK They may be entitled to limited financial help from the authorities She is entitled to free NHS treatment
Refugee	A woman who, owing to a well-founded fear of being persecuted for reasons of race, religion, nationality, membership of a particular social group, or political opinion, is outside the country of her nationality and is unable to or unwilling to avail herself of the protection of that country	The woman has proven to the authorities that their asylum claim is valid She has the same legal rights as British citizens She can work, study and claim state benefits She is entitled to free NHS treatment
Failed asylum seeker	A woman whose asylum claim has been refused by the Home Office must return to her home country	She has the right to appeal against the decision but if unsuccessful, must leave the UK She has no legal rights to work, study or claim benefits in the UK while awaiting a decision She is entitled to limited NHS treatment

Reproduced with permission from Asif, S., Baugh, A., Jones, N.W., 2015. The obstetric care of asylum seekers and refugee women in the UK. *Obstet. Gynaecol.* 17 (4), 223–231.

seeking and refused asylum often do not know what they are entitled to and are not given enough information (in a form they can understand) on how to access NHS healthcare and the function of specific healthcare services (Higginbottom et al., 2019).

The literature demonstrates that some of these barriers affect women refused asylum more acutely. For example, the treatment being withheld because of healthcare entitlement policies, people avoiding services because of fears about the cost or being reported to the Home Office, greater financial difficulties because many people refused asylum cannot claim public funds and are not allowed to work (Nellums et al., 2018).

Not only do refugee and asylum-seeking women frequently lack knowledge of sexual and reproductive health services, but they may also not have had health education regarding the importance of such services (WHO, 2015). It is clear that refugees and asylum seekers are not a homogenous group but are differentiated by cultural norms, education and past experiences. This diversity is evident in their social and sexual health backgrounds, such as the experience of FGM and varied levels of contraceptives, STI and screening knowledge (Sudbury and Robinson, 2016). Several initiatives have been set up in the UK to promote reproductive health knowledge among migrants by refugee community organisations, health professionals and schools (Wilson et al., 2007). They include antenatal classes specifically developed for pregnant refugee and asylum-seeking women (McCarthy et al., 2013).

Maternity services should always be classified as 'urgent' and 'immediately necessary' and therefore not subject to upfront charging. However, evidence has been found that they have been withheld from pregnant women who have been refused asylum and were unable to pay (Maternity Action and Refugee Council, 2013).

Evidence suggests that moving people seeking asylum between accommodations under the Home Office dispersal policy can cause particular problems by interrupting their care. One study found this was a barrier to HIV care in England, leading to late access to services, compromised care and increased transmission (Creighton et al., 2004). Pregnant women who are entitled to support in England and Scotland have experienced interruptions and delays in getting both antenatal and routine healthcare at their dispersal destination (Maternity Action and Refugee Council, 2013; Da Lomba et al., 2014).

According to Maternity Action and the Refugee Council (2013), dispersal results in poorer pregnancy and maternal health outcomes for women seeking asylum than other pregnant women. Dispersal not only affects the continuity of care, but it can also leave a woman isolated from friends and family and mean services are not joined up, so both women and children are 'vulnerable to gaps and oversights'. It is often left to charities and voluntary organisations to fill these gaps.

When dispersal occurs late in pregnancy, it adds to other complex health needs a woman seeking asylum may face (such as sexual and psychosocial challenges, infectious diseases, female genital mutilation, destitution) and exacerbates the already elevated rates of maternal and child mortality and morbidity in this population (Asif et al., 2015).

Practice Point

You should be aware of the rights of refugees and asylum seekers. You must recognise the struggles of women in these situations. The midwife has a legal and professional responsibility to provide care to all pregnant women in the first instance and not act as a gatekeeper to maternity service. The next section discusses the role the midwife may play in creating barriers to pregnancy care.

The Midwife as a Barrier

Previous chapters have discussed the importance of cultural awareness as a key skill for midwives, which leads to the acquirement of other skills essential to develop cultural competency. However, there are other barriers created by a midwife, either consciously or unconsciously, for women requiring culturally competent care. There may be too much of an expectation by health professionals that women and their families will adapt to the dominant culture, rather than the maternity service being responsive and sensitive to the needs of a multicultural population (Henderson et al., 2013).

STEREOTYPING AND UNCONSCIOUS BIAS

The barriers created by midwives are several and, at times, not recognised as an important aspect for women's satisfaction with maternity care. Midwives are the main healthcare professionals in a woman's pregnancy and hence, have regular contact during care provision. The attitudes of maternity care healthcare providers are critical determinants of care; factors of stereotyping, racism, unconscious bias and direct and indirect discrimination create barriers to women accessing and engaging with care (Higginbottom et al., 2019).

Stereotyping is a fixed, overgeneralised belief about a particular group or class of people. By stereotyping, we infer that a person has a whole range of characteristics and abilities that we assume all group members have. Stereotypes are learned, explicit or implicit and are taught to people by social influences (Rosenthal et al., 2016). Explicit stereotyping refers to beliefs held by a person to make a judgement, whilst implicit stereotyping are assumptions made subconsciously by a person, of which they have no control or awareness. There is no doubt of the role that stereotyping plays in ethnocentric attitudes (Chakkarath, 2010). Unfortunately, stereotypes can be negative or positive; for example, all women can cook or are poor drivers. No social group is homogenous, so stereotyping means that there may be a misrepresentation of individuals from that group. Stereotyping creates prejudice, leading to attitudes of treating a woman in a particular way because of assumptions of categorising her to a group of people. Women may be treated depending on stereotyping, which can lead to inappropriate care and impact an optimum pregnancy outcome. Stereotypes control our social judgements and may create emotional distance between you and women from different cultures.

Stereotype threat refers to the anxieties and expectations that can be activated in stigmatised groups when negative stereotypes about their group are made. This can lead to increased anxiety and impaired decision making, which can lead to unhealthy behaviours, poor communication from women to midwives, lower levels of adherence to medical advice, increased blood pressure and weight gain among stigmatised groups (Aronson et al., 2013; Spencer et al., 2016; Williams and Mohammed, 2013).

Simply put, unconscious bias is prejudice in favour of or against a person or group of people. You may fail to see that you are biased when caring for women from different cultures. It is difficult to recognise unconscious bias, which requires a constant commitment to making a difference (Bucknor-Ferron and Zagaja, 2016). However, midwives are human, and it is inherent they provide care that is affected by unconscious bias. Biases are either conscious (explicit) or unconscious (implicit). **Unconscious bias** may result in quick judgements that may not be logical to others; it is based on our own background, culture and personal experiences and often originates at a very early age (Cuellar, 2017). An organisation's **unconscious bias** is embedded in how policies and procedures are developed; if an organisation is truly unbiased, the attributes, characteristics and behaviours of all the organisation members will result in feeling included and promoted (Cuellar, 2017).

Microaggression is a word used to describe everyday subtle remarks or actions that are insulting to marginalised groups. Microaggressions are often the result of unconscious biases that lead to unintended discrimination against or degradation of socially marginalised people in a society, whether by race, gender, sexual orientation, age, language, origin, religion, disability or any other characteristic (Bellack, 2015).

Bucknor-Ferron and Zagaja (2016) suggest five strategies to eliminate unconscious bias. You can use these strategies to reflect on your personal biases and determine how these can be reduced or limited in your midwifery practice.

Five Strategies to Eliminate Unconscious Bias

Strategy	Rationale
• **Personal awareness**	A process of looking inward to recognise beliefs and values that can lead to unconscious bias; acquiring personal awareness requires an internal compass used to guide daily interactions. This compass can help midwives recognise acceptable and unacceptable attitudes and behaviours.
• **Recognition**	Forces midwives to constantly look inward and create an awareness of how others perceive them.
• **Empathy**	Most midwives naturally have a sense of empathy, but some women and situations can raise a barrier to empathy. For example, caring for women who participate in risk-taking behaviours that result in adverse health outcomes can make it more difficult for a midwife to be empathetic. Refusing to acknowledge this emotional necessity can produce negative outcomes during patient interactions and care.

Continued

Five Strategies to Eliminate Unconscious Bias – cont'd	
Strategy	**Rationale**
• **Advocacy**	Support for women as they navigate a complex healthcare system is called advocacy. In the presence of unconscious bias, midwives' advocacy can support women to receive the individualised care they need.
• **Education**	Enhanced knowledge is central to raising awareness, recognising unconscious bias and reducing its prevalence. Education that focuses on sensitivity and the existence of unconscious bias in healthcare facilities.

Adapted from Bucknor-Ferron, P., Zagaja, L., 2016. Five strategies to combat unconscious bias. *Nursing 2020.* 46 (11), 61–62.

Practice Point

Being aware that stereotyping and unconscious bias are present in maternity services is the first step to changing attitudes that impact women's care. You should recognise beliefs and values that can lead to unconscious bias. If you observe microaggressions, you should challenge them. More importantly, if women express a concern that they are being treated differently, then you should heed their views and escalate the concern.

RACIAL DISCRIMINATION

There have been many reports where ethnic minority women have stated being treated unfairly due to their ethnicity, language or culture (Henderson et al., 2013; Higginbottom et al., 2019; McLeish and Redshaw, 2019). Midwives will always state that they treat all women fairly and facilitate inclusivity; however, it is the woman who determines they are being treated differently. Racist behaviour is often used to explain the reason for this negative treatment. There are many definitions provided for racism, one being that it is the negative attitude behind behaviour that assumes that the other person is not as valuable, that they are not as 'worthy' (Cross-Sudworth, 2007). This suggests that racism is difficult to prove, and herein lies the issue when a woman reports negative behaviour because they must first confirm that it is due to a negative attitude. Racism is the belief that personality, behaviour and morals can be traced back to race and the belief that one race is superior to another as opposed to discrimination, which is acting on racist thoughts. Racism is also defined as unfair and preventable disparities in power, resources, capacities or opportunities centred on ethnic, racial, religious or cultural differences (Berman and Paradies, 2010). Hence, women may be treated differently due to their race or ethnic background and, more importantly, be denied appropriate care because they are deemed inferior.

Power is a necessary precondition for racial discrimination, as it depends on the ability to give or withhold social benefits, facilities, services, opportunities, etc., from someone who should be entitled to them, and are denied based on race, colour or national origin (Randall, 2019). Racial discrimination is present in everyday life, although if raised as a concern is most likely to be met with denial that it occurs. Women who have experienced discrimination in the past may be more reluctant to seek healthcare, as they may perceive it as a setting of increased risk for discrimination (i.e. refusal of service or lower quality of care) (Rivenbark and Ichou, 2020). Therefore, a barrier is created by midwives who racially discriminate against women based on their ethnicity or race.

Debates have been raised about racism caused by cultural differences rather than biological differences such as skin colour. Cultural racism is a concept applied to prejudice and discrimination based on cultural differences between different racial groups. Cultural racism can lead to unconscious bias at an individual level and can lead to discrimination. In addition, cultural racism relies on stereotyping that leads to unconscious bias and has a detrimental effect on health (Razai et al., 2021). In clinical encounters, these processes lead to women who are culturally different to the majority culture receiving inferior pregnancy care. In addition, negative experiences within a culturally insensitive healthcare service may create barriers, inhibit access to healthcare and influence healthcare seeking behaviours among ethnic minority groups (Public Health England, 2020).

Most interventions aimed at reducing cultural racism focus on addressing implicit biases or enhancing cultural competence. A recent review found that cultural competency interventions can lead to improvements in provider knowledge, skills and attitudes regarding culture and healthcare access and utilisation, but little evidence indicates that these interventions affect health outcomes and health equity (Truong et al., 2014).

Practice Point

You should be aware that everyone has unconscious biases. It is important to reflect on your unconscious biases regularly. This reflection will reduce the likelihood of the care you provide impacting negatively on the woman. There should be zero tolerance for racism and discrimination in maternity services. The crucial point is that all racist and discriminatory behaviour should be challenged and stopped.

Barriers in Maternity Services
WHAT ARE THE BARRIERS?

Although maternity units attempt to provide maternity care that caters for a diverse childbearing population, women face many barriers before they can access care. As previously discussed, this ranges from lack of knowledge of how maternity services work and how to access maternity care to organisational and professional factors. A study found that for black and minority ethnic women, asylum seekers and refugees, language barriers and unfamiliarity with the UK system had the biggest impact on how care was accessed, engaged with and how they experienced their maternity care (Rayment-Jones et al., 2019). Policies and guidance have been developed to improve these issues; however, another issue arises with women engaging with maternity services once access is gained.

Other matters that women face when there is access and engagement with maternity services are culturally unsafe services, lack of cultural competency, discrimination, racism, stereotyping and unconscious bias. As observed by some professionals, the maternity system in the UK has been designed for a homogenous pregnancy experience and a static population (Phillimore, 2015). This system does not work for migrant women or women from ethnic minority groups and is a fact UK maternity services recognise. Maternity services in the UK continue to struggle to provide appropriate care that meets the needs of women from diverse populations (Puthussery, 2016; Knight et al., 2016). The result of decades of marginalisation of minority ethnic welfare issues has highlighted the need for culturally sensitive and specific services in health authorities with diverse populations (Phillimore, 2015).

Quality of care (QoC) has been recognised as being pivotal in reducing maternal and infant mortality and morbidity. The WHO (2021) definition of quality of care is 'the extent to which healthcare services provided to individuals and patient populations improve desired health outcomes'. WHO (2021) has developed quality standards for maternal and newborn health as a guideline for what quality standards should consist and how they can be achieved (Table 5.4).

The WHO also provides a framework of organisational management strategies to improve quality of care (Fig. 5.2) to help the healthcare system achieve its desired goals (WHO, 2006).

This is a general framework that suggests that overall, the health systems should focus on improving six domains of organisational management strategies to improve QoC – information, leadership, engagement with patients and population, use of regulation and standards, developing

---

TABLE 5.4 ■ Developing Quality Standards for Maternal and Newborn Care

Safe–Delivering healthcare that minimises risks and harm to service users, including avoiding preventable injuries and reducing medical errors.

Effective–Providing services based on scientific knowledge and evidence-based guidelines.

Timely–Reducing delays in providing and receiving healthcare.

Efficient–Delivering healthcare in a manner that maximises resource use and avoids waste.

Equitable–Delivering healthcare that does not differ in quality according to personal characteristics such as gender, race, ethnicity, geographical location or socioeconomic status.

People-centred–Providing care that takes into account the preferences and aspirations of individual service users and the culture of their community.

From World Health Organization, 2021. Developing quality standards for maternal and newborn care. https://www.who.int/maternal_child_adolescent/topics/quality-of-care/en/.

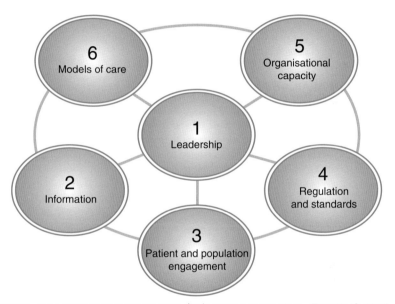

Fig. 5.2 Organisational management strategies to improve quality of care (From WHO, 2006).

organisational capacity and models of care (WHO, 2006). These domains are relevant to improving access for diverse women, particularly information, engagement, use of regulation and standards and models of care.

ENGAGEMENT WITH WOMEN

Women from different cultures have many issues when trying to access maternity care. Currently, maternity units provide one system of accessing maternity care, usually via a general practitioner (GP). However, government guidance has recommended that women could self-refer to maternity care Department of Health (DOH), 2007). Women may not wish to access care or may find it difficult to access care via their GP. There may be gender-based restrictions related to culture, such as no access to a female GP or not attending appointments unless accompanied by a male member of their family. Hence, women may choose to wait rather than be seen by a man or until they can be accompanied by a suitable person, keeping in accordance with their cultural values.

The NHS needs to organise its services around women and families. Community hubs should be identified to help every woman access the services they need, with obstetric units providing care if they need more specialised services (National Maternity Review, 2016). The concept of a community hub is a local centre where women can access various elements of their maternity care. They could be in a children's centre or a freestanding midwifery unit. Hubs, hospitals and other services should work together to wrap the care around each woman (National Maternity Review, 2016).

Access issues can be solved by creating direct access to maternity care and making this access easy and stress-free. Most Trusts allow a woman to self-refer for maternity care or via a GP referral. However, the woman is expected to complete a form by hand or online, which will be difficult for women who are not computer literate or have a language barrier. Some Trusts have a dedicated self-referral line where an administrative person can take the woman's details over the phone to complete a referral. These strategies are geared towards women who do not have a language barrier. Other women who cannot self-refer have no choice but to resort to attending a GP appointment. GPs who cannot offer interpreting services for appointments may impact women unless they can attend with someone who speaks English. If the woman does not wish to reveal her pregnancy too early, this may impact when she can schedule a GP appointment which may be given 1 to 2 weeks later, and those women who delay revealing their pregnancy for cultural reasons results in further delay in accessing maternity care.

INFORMATION AVAILABILITY

Women who do not have access to timely information cannot negotiate maternity services and understand how their pregnancy will be managed and their options. There is insufficient information about services or health promotion materials in different languages or media formats. Although providers attempt to provide appropriate information for all women, rapid population changes with newer migrant groups appearing in some areas mean it is difficult to ensure inclusivity (Cha, 2013). Internet access is also not available to every woman, and if there are reduced facilities for computer access such as libraries, information about maternity services which is mainly on the internet, is further restricted. Women from different cultures also face barriers if they are unable to procure information in usual formats. This is particularly relevant to women who are marginalised or who have language or literacy barriers. Policymakers and advocacy groups have highlighted the neglect of effective communication strategies to provide information through community or faith groups to reach those less likely to proactively (Cha, 2013). In incidences, some mothers have been processed through an impersonal system with lack of regard to their needs, with staff not realising their information needs about the purpose and operation of the maternity system and the progress of their pregnancies (McLeish and Redshaw, 2019).

Practice Point

The realisation of barriers that women can face when trying to access or engage with maternity services is one to take heed of. You may have seen this or be aware of this in your clinical practice. Therefore, flexibility is needed for the woman you know may be struggling with accessing or engaging with services. This could be as simple as providing alternative ways for a woman to register for maternity care and going the extra step to provide appropriate health advice.

MODELS OF CARE

It has been recommended that cultural factors should be taken into account in the planning and delivery of services to effectively encourage service uptake as an important step in reducing maternal and newborn mortality (WHO, 2003). Hence, maternity services should focus on ensuring that models of care incorporate the cultural needs. Ideally, a model of care should be created that caters for a diverse woman. Unfortunately, this is not the case, and a 'one size fits all' model, despite its high standards, may not meet the needs of women from diverse backgrounds (McFadden et al., 2013).

Women with diverse needs struggle with maternity services when their cultural needs are not catered for. Models of maternity care need to be designed to meet the needs of all women in society to ensure equitable access to services and address health inequalities (Fair et al., 2020). There are only a few examples of innovative approaches for maternity care provision from some areas with a high population density of migrants to address the health needs of vulnerable and socially disadvantaged women (Puthussery, 2016).

You should be aware that a woman may see a different midwife at each antenatal appointment, another midwife during labour and yet another midwife postnatally. This model of care impacts women engaging with maternity services and reduces the ability to form a relationship and gain trust and relationship. Women may struggle with this type of care and may find it difficult to maintain their cultural values leading to a decision to not engage with care; the WHO supports the notion of 'culturally appropriate' maternity care services that take into account a woman's personal preferences and their cultural and value system (WHO, 2003). However, studies have found that factors that affected access or utilisation of maternity care preference for local services that are either unavailable and/or inaccessible, lack of joined-up services and difficulty in navigating through the services, inability to access information, perceived impersonal and insensitive nature of the health system (Hollowell et al., 2012). Women have reported that they see too many midwives and doctors throughout their pregnancy and birth and do not always know who they are and what their role is. For some women, this leads to confusion, and they cannot build up a rapport with healthcare professionals (National Maternity Review, 2016).

Continuity of carer is one model that has been at the centre of maternity policy in the UK since Changing Childbirth (DOH, 1993) and the emphasis on choice, continuity and control for all women. Better Births (National Maternity Review, 2016) has also put forward continuity of carer as a key element to increase woman's satisfaction with maternity services. The aim of having a named midwife caring for women through pregnancy is needed by a culturally diverse woman. There is evidence of improved access to care by women who find services hard to reach and better coordination of care with specialist and obstetric services (Royal College of Midwives (RCM), 2018). Continuity of carer can significantly improve outcomes for women from ethnic minorities and those living in deprived areas (Rayment-Jones et al., 2019; Homer et al., 2017; RCM, 2018). However, the availability of continuity of carer model in maternity services is limited. Hence, barriers are created for women due to care provision not being conducive to individual and culturally sensitive care.

Exercise

Review the following scenario regarding a woman's experience of pregnancy.

Safah booked for her first pregnancy at 12 weeks. Since then, she has seen a different midwife at each antenatal appointment. Safah has had concerns about the delivery and where this will be as she has no other family apart from her husband in the UK. She had discussed this in an early antenatal appointment but has not seen the midwife she spoke to since. Safah now feels there is no point discussing her needs about the birth as she knows this will not be the midwife who delivers her baby.

Learning Activity

1. How do you think this experience will impact Safah engaging with maternity service?
2. What do you think could be the key solution for Safah to improve her confidence in receiving care?
3. Think about your clinical practice and whether this care delivery is the usual practice.

LACK OF PRACTICE GUIDANCE

Maternity services are responsible for guiding midwives on ensuring that each woman is cared for in a culturally sensitive way. Lack of clear definitions and practical guidance has been found to leave healthcare professionals uncertain regarding how they might address cultural and religious needs, alongside delivering effective clinical care (Sartori, 2010). Some maternity units have limited guidance around these issues, but most policies on care provision focus on direct midwives' care, not how the care should be delivered. Differences between the cultures of healthcare services and service users have been recognised as a major issue in service delivery (Coast et al., 2014). Therefore, guidance is needed that specially addresses care delivery.

It has been recommended that cultural factors should be taken into account in the planning and delivery of services to effectively encourage service uptake as an important step in reducing maternal and newborn mortality (WHO, 2003). Maternity services should provide access to basic information about maternal, perinatal and reproductive health; and care-seeking targeted at women, families, communities and providers, as well as a commitment to humanised services (Coast et al., 2014). Even if there is guidance available, there is no evaluation of how this is used in practice. Maternity services need to ensure that the organisational culture does not subjugate midwifery (for example, a culture of obstetric interventions) and allows different cultures of practice to work in equal partnership to reduce barriers to practising 'proper' midwifery care (Frith et al., 2014). Unfortunately, barriers are perpetuated by health services that do not communicate effectively or offer culturally appropriate care (Pangas et al., 2019). Organisational culture is seen as problematic and it has been found that midwives may become a less powerful sub-culture, preventing individualised midwifery care (Frith et al., 2014).

Learning Activity

You should think about the culture in your maternity unit and whether your policies explicitly consider the cultural needs of the women you are caring for. If so, you can think about how this translates to direct midwifery care. Can you think of any examples that involve a midwife considering the woman's cultural needs when providing prescribed midwifery care?

LACK OF CULTURAL COMPETENCY TRAINING

There is a need for midwives to have regular access to cultural competency and cultural safety training. Many maternity units do not offer cultural training as part of midwives' yearly mandatory training. If cultural competency training is provided, this may not be offered in great focus but as a thread through sessions. Cultural competency training extends far beyond the understanding of language needs and lists of 'dos' and 'do nots' or facts about other value systems but should incorporate helping midwives to create an atmosphere where all women feel able to express and discuss their specific healthcare needs (Hassan et al., 2020). Cultural competence education that does not incorporate these essential elements has been criticised in the literature as perpetuating cultural stereotypes (Hoke and Robbins, 2011; Clark et al., 2011).

Cultural competence training can include understanding the central role of culture in all lives and how it shapes behaviour respect and acceptance of cultural differences, learning to effectively utilise culturally adapted and culturally specific practices and continuous development of one's awareness of personal cultural influences and prejudices or biases (Hark and DeLisser, 2011; Purnell and Paulanka, 1998, 2012). Cultural competence training has mostly focused on developing knowledge, attitudes, awareness and sensitivity of healthcare workers. However, the literature reiterates the need to reach further than this and focus on teaching the skills needed to translate knowledge and awareness into tangible practitioner behaviours that can be consistently applied and assessed in healthcare encounters and settings (Hark and DeLisser, 2011; Dreachslin et al., 2012).

Cultural sensitivity from midwives plays a fundamental role in women's experience of care. A lack of cultural awareness on the part of health services or professionals prevents cultural beliefs and practices from being recognised as legitimate and significant (Russo et al., 2015; Shafiei et al., 2012; Wojnar, 2015). Professionals have confessed lack of knowledge about the complex lives of migrant women. Midwives who lack cultural sensitivity inadvertently create a barrier to the woman by not exploring her cultural views of pregnancy.

USE OF INTERPRETERS

Language barriers have already been cited as a barrier to effective care and, lack of access to trained interpreters continues to be a problem. Midwives have revealed concern at not having 24-hour access to translators or interpreters because these were an expensive resource; hospital translators were often difficult to access in person or by phone, especially out of normal working hours (Tobin and Murphy-Lawless, 2014). Hence, women are unable to understand aspects of their care and, equally as important, unable to express their wishes and desires regarding their pregnancy.

Although it is recommended to provide interpreters for women who cannot speak English and not use family members or friends (CEMACH, 2011), problems exist in the provision of these services. Issues include failure of the interpreters to attend appointments or their inability to understand medical terminology, failure from professionals to book interpretation services, lack of interpreters for speaking uncommon languages and unsuitable use of family members to interpret (McClure et al., 2011; Phillimore, 2015). Maternity services need to have a more robust way of ensuring that women with language barriers are highlighted at the first access to services and that appropriate strategies are in place to support their language needs. Some midwives have reported that face-to-face interpreters are not always available out of hours and often must be booked 24 hours in advance, which is often not feasible in the maternity setting (Maternity Action, 2018).

Alternatives have been made by maternity services to provide both face to face and telephone interpretation services. However, these are not ideal for certain elements of pregnancy care, such as during labour or in emergencies. Effective interpretation services can reduce the barriers women face in expressing their wishes and having informed choices during pregnancy and childbirth. However, for maternity units that do not offer this facility, the danger is that women may go through pregnancy experiencing care that is not individualised and culturally sensitive. In addition, the ability to access and engage with maternity care is severely impacted and may lead to poorer pregnancy outcomes.

Exercise

Review the following scenario regarding barriers to accessing care.

A Somali woman named Farah is having her fourth child and has already been to her GP to arrange a referral to her local hospital. There was a delay with the GP in sending her referral letter. She had been posted a booking appointment for 4 weeks when she would be 16 weeks. Farah and her husband do not speak English very well, and an interpreter has not been arranged at her booking appointment. The GP had failed to notify the hospital that Farah and her husband do not speak good English. Subsequently, the appointment must be rearranged for when she is 19 weeks, nearly halfway through her pregnancy.

Learning Activity

After reading this scenario, think about the barriers in maternity services that have delayed access to care for Farah. How could these barriers have been avoided, and how could this be prevented from happening in the future? In your maternity unit, are there issues with women booking late? If so, were steps taken to find out why?

The following information provides some strategies that can be used to increase women's access and engagement with maternity services.

WHAT STEPS CAN BE TAKEN TO IMPROVE ACCESS?

Individual Steps

- Beware of language barriers, offer an interpreter at the first instance.
- Never assume how a woman may behave if they are from a certain cultural background.
- Adopt the habit of asking pertinent questions about a woman's beliefs before planning care.
- Be supportive and willing to discuss any cultural norms with the woman in a non-biased manner, for example, wearing certain clothes, obeying rituals, need for chaperones and discussing sexual health with a male professional.
- It would be useful to find out how pregnancy care is carried out in the woman's country of origin to correct any misconceptions. Discuss with the woman how the healthcare system works in the UK, for example, the pattern of care, blood tests, seeing the GP etc.

Organisational Steps

- Adopting culturally appropriate advice leaflets, maternity notes for a woman regarding pregnancy, for example, on diet, breastfeeding and postnatal care.
- Cultural knowledge packs for health professionals available in ward areas as quick reference guides.
- Adopting the use of community centres to provide information on certain cultures as a regular occurrence. For example, training of new staff, devising of information packs for women.
- Use culture as the first point of assessment for the woman when devising care plans or patterns of care. This will allow consideration for acknowledging cultural norms or respecting any taboos.

Practice Point

You can help women engage with healthcare services by using culturally appropriate posters and literature to target particular groups. However, maintaining engagement with certain groups can be achieved by ensuring that culturally sensitive care and advice are given. Creating an understanding with women can be achieved by acknowledging cultural differences and at the same time facilitating woman's needs by removing barriers that may compromise their culture.

REFLECTIVE QUESTIONS

1. How do the barriers that women experience relate to your maternity unit?
2. Do you think some of the individual barriers that women face are a relevant issue in midwifery practice?
3. How can issues of racism and discrimination be addressed in your maternity services?
4. Why do you think that stigma may be particularly difficult for some women to overcome?

References

All Party Parliamentary Group on Refugees, 2017. Refugees welcome? The experience of new refugees in the UK: a report by the All Party Parliamentary Group On Refugees. Available at: https://reliefweb.int/report/world/refugees-welcome-experience-new-refugees-uk-report-all-party-parliamentary-group.

Aronson, J., Burgess, D., Phelan, S.M., Juarez, L., 2013. Unhealthy interactions: the role of stereotype threat in health disparities. Am. J. Public Health 103 (1), 50–56.

Asadi, L., Amiri, F., Safinejad, H., 2020. Investigating the effect of health literacy level on improving the quality of care during pregnancy in pregnant women covered by health centers. J. Educ Health Promot. 9, 286.

Asif, S., Baugh, A., Jones, N.W., 2015. The obstetric care of asylum seekers and refugee women in the UK. Obstet. Gynaecol. 17 (4), 223–231.

Babatunde, T., Moreno-Leguizamon, C.J., 2012. Daily and cultural issues of postnatal depression in African women immigrants in South East London: tips for health professionals. Nurs. Res. Pract. 2012, 181640.

Bellack, J.P., 2015. Unconscious bias: an obstacle to cultural competence. J. Nurs. Educ. 54 (9), S63–S64.

Berman, G., Paradies, Y., 2010. Racism, disadvantage and multiculturalism: towards effective anti-racist praxis. Ethn. Racial Stud. 33 (2), 214–232.

Bracke, P., Delaruelle, K., Verhaeghe, M., 2019. Dominant cultural and personal stigma beliefs and the utilization of mental health services: a cross-national comparison. Front. Sociol. 4, 40.

Bradby, H., Humphris, R., Newall, D., Phillimore, J., 2015. Public Health Aspects of Migrant Health: A Review of the Evidence on Health Status for Refugees and Asylum Seekers in the European Region. WHO Regional Office for Europe, Copenhagen.

Briscoe, L., Lavender, T., 2009. Exploring maternity care for asylum seekers and refugees. Br. J. Midwifery 17 (1), 17–23.

Bucknor-Ferron, P., Zagaja, L., 2016. Five strategies to combat unconscious bias. Nursing 2020 46 (11), 61–62.

Carolan, M., Cassar, L., 2010. Antenatal care perceptions of pregnant African women attending maternity services in Melbourne, Australia. Midwifery 26 (2), 189–201.

CEMACH, 2011. Saving mothers' lives: reviewing maternal deaths to make motherhood safer: 2006–2008. BJOG. 118, s1–203.

Cha, E., 2013. Inequalities and Multiple Discrimination in Access to and Quality of Healthcare. European Union Agency for Fundamental Rights, Luxembourg. 3–107.

Chakkarath, P., 2010. Stereotypes in social psychology: the west-east differentiation as a reflection of western traditions of thought. Psychological Studies. 55 (1), 18–25.

Clark, L., Calvillo, E., Dela Cruz, F., Fongwa, M., Kools, S., Lowe, J., Mastel-Smith, B., 2011. Cultural competencies for graduate nursing education. J Prof. Nurs. 27 (3), 133–139.

Coast, E., Jones, E., Portela, A., Lattof, S.R., 2014. Maternity care services and culture: a systematic global mapping of interventions. PloS one 9 (9), e108130.

Copeland, D., 2019. Respectful maternity care charter. White Ribbon Alliance. Available at: https://www.whiteribbonalliance.org/respectful-maternity-care-charter/.

Creighton, S., Sethi, G., Edwards, S.G., Miller, R., 2004. Dispersal of HIV positive asylum seekers: national survey of UK healthcare providers. BMJ. 329 (7461), 322–323.

Cross-Sudworth, F., 2007. Racism and discrimination in maternity services. Br. J. Midwifery 15 (6), 327–331.

Cuellar, N.G., 2017. Unconscious bias: What is yours? J. Transcult. Nurs. 28 (4), 333.

Da Lomba, S., 2014. Vulnerability, irregular migrants' health-related rights and the European court of human rights. Eur. J. Health Law. 21 (4), 339–364.

Das, A.K., Olfson, M., McCurtis, H.L., Weissman, M.M., 2006. Depression in African Americans: breaking barriers to detection and treatment: community-based studies tend to ignore high-risk groups of African Americans. J. Fam. Pract. 55 (1), 30–40.

Department of Health (DOH), 1993. Changing Childbirth. Part 1: Report of the Expert Maternity Group. Department of Health, London, United Kingdom.

Department of Health (DOH), 2007. Maternity matters: choice, access and continuity of care in a safe service. Available at: https://dera.ioe.ac.uk/9429/7/dh_074199_Redacted.pdf

Dreachslin, J.L., Gilbert, M.J., Malone, B., 2012. Diversity and Cultural Competence in Health Care: a Systems Approach. John Wiley & Sons, Hoboken, NJ.

Fair, F., Raben, L., Watson, H., Vivilaki, V., van den Muijsenbergh, M., Soltani, H., ORAMMA team, 2020. Migrant women's experiences of pregnancy, childbirth and maternity care in European countries: A systematic review. PloS one 15 (2), e0228378.

Feldman, R., 2013. When maternity doesn't matter: dispersing pregnant women seeking asylum. Reprod. Health Matters 21 (42), 212–217.

Frith, L., Sinclair, M., Vehviläinen-Julkunen, K., Beeckman, K., Lotyved, C., Luybens, A., 2014. Organisational culture in maternity care: a scoping review. Evid. Based Midwifery 12 (1) 16–2.

Gilbert, P., Gilbert, J., Sanghera, J., 2004. A focus group exploration of the impact of izzat, shame, subordination and entrapment on mental health and service use in South Asian women living in Derby. Ment. Health Relig. Cult 7 (2), 109–130.

Hark, L., DeLisser, H. (Eds.), 2011. Achieving Cultural Competency: A Case-Based Approach to Training Health Professionals. John Wiley & Sons, Oxford.

Hassan, S.M., Leavey, C., Rooney, J.S., Puthussery, S., 2020. A qualitative study of healthcare professionals' experiences of providing maternity care for Muslim women in the UK. BMC Pregnancy Childbirth 20 (1), 1–10.

Henderson, J., Gao, H., Redshaw, M., 2013. Experiencing maternity care: the care received and perceptions of women from different ethnic groups. BMC Pregnancy Childbirth. 13 (1), 1–14.

Higginbottom, G.M., Morgan, M., Alexandre, M., Chiu, Y., Forgeron, J., Kocay, D., Barolia, R., 2015. Immigrant women's experiences of maternity-care services in Canada: a systematic review using a narrative synthesis. Syst Rev 11 (4), 1–113.

Higginbottom, G.M.A., Evans, C., Morgan, M., Bharj, K.K., Eldridge, J., Hussain, B., 2019. Experience of and access to maternity care in the UK by immigrant women: a narrative synthesis systematic review. BMJ Open 9 (12), e029478.

Hill, N., Hunt, E., Hyrkäs, K., 2012. Somali immigrant women's health care experiences and beliefs regarding pregnancy and birth in the United States. J. Transcult. Nurs. 23 (1), 72–81.

Hoban, E., Liamputtong, P., 2013. Cambodian migrant women's postpartum experiences in Victoria, Australia. Midwifery 29 (7), 772–778.

Hoke, M.M., Robbins, L.K., 2011. Continuing the cultural competency journey through exploration of knowledge, attitudes, and skills with advanced practice psychiatric nursing students: an exemplar. Nursing Clinics. 46 (2), 201–205.

Hollowell, J., Oakley, L., Vigurs, C., Barnett-Page, E., Kavanagh, J., Oliver, S., 2012. Increasing the Early Initiation of Antenatal Care by Black and Minority Ethnic Women in the United Kingdom: A Systematic Review and Mixed Methods Synthesis of Women's Views and the Literature on Intervention Effectiveness. Social Science Research Unit, Institute of Education, University of London.

Homer, C.S., Leap, N., Edwards, N., Sandall, J., 2017. Midwifery continuity of carer in an area of high socio-economic disadvantage in London: a retrospective analysis of Albany Midwifery Practice outcomes using routine data (1997–2009). Midwifery. 48, 1–10.

Hughson, J.A., Marshall, F., Daly, J.O., Woodward-Kron, R., Hajek, J., Story, D., 2018. Health professionals' views on health literacy issues for culturally and linguistically diverse women in maternity care: barriers, enablers and the need for an integrated approach. Aust. Health Rev. 42 (1), 10–20.

Keygnaert, I., Ivanova, O., Guieu, A., Van Parys, A., Leye, E., Roelens, K., 2016. What is the evidence on the reduction of inequalities in accessibility and quality of maternal health care delivery for migrants? A review of the existing evidence in the WHO European region. World Health Organization, Regional, Copenhagen.

Knight, M., Bunch, K., Tuffnell, D., Shakespeare, J., Kotnis, R., Kenyon, S., Kurinczuk, J.J., 2019. Saving Lives, Improving Mothers' Care: Lessons Learned to Inform Maternity Care from the UK and Ireland Confidential Enquiries into Maternal Deaths and Morbidity 2015–17. MBRRACE-UK, Oxford.

Lillrank, A., 2015. Trust, Vacillation and Neglect: Refugee women's experiences regarding pregnancy and birth giving in Finland. Nord. J. Migr. Res. 5 (2), 83–89.

Lindquist, A., Kurinczuk, J.J., Redshaw, M., Knight, M., 2015. Experiences, utilisation and outcomes of maternity care in England among women from different socio-economic groups: findings from the 2010 National Maternity Survey. BJOG 122 (12), 1610–1617.

Link, B.G., Phelan, J.C., 2001. Conceptualizing stigma. Annu. Rev. Sociol. 27 (1), 363–385.

Maternity Action and Refugee Council, 2013. When maternity doesn't matter. Available at: https://www.maternityaction.org.uk/wp-content/uploads/2013/09/When_Maternity_Doesn_t_Matter_-_Ref_Council-Maternity_Action_report_Feb2013.pdf.

Maternity Action, 2018. Mothers' voices, exploring experiences of maternity and health in low income women and children from diverse ethnic backgrounds. Available at: https://www.maternityaction.org.uk/wp-content/uploads/MothersVoices2018-FINAL.pdf.

McCarthy, R., Winder, V., Newburn, M., 2013. Facilitating Antenatal Courses Attended by Asylum Seekers and Refugees. NCT, London.

McClure, J.H., Cooper, G.M., Clutton-Brock, T.H., Centre for Maternal and Child Enquiries, 2011. Saving mothers' lives: reviewing maternal deaths to make motherhood safer: 2006–8: a review. Br. J. Anaesth. 107 (2), 127–132.

McConville, B., 2014. Respectful maternity care–how the UK is learning from the developing world. Midwifery 30 (2), 154–157.

McFadden, A., Renfrew, M.J., Atkin, K., 2013. Does cultural context make a difference to women's experiences of maternity care? A qualitative study comparing the perspectives of breast-feeding women of Bangladeshi origin and health practitioners. Health Expect. 16 (4), e124–e135.

McKnight, P., Goodwin, L., Kenyon, S., 2019. A systematic review of asylum-seeking women's views and experiences of UK maternity care. Midwifery 77, 16–23.

McLeish, J., Alliance, M., 2002. Mothers in Exile. The Maternity Alliance, London.

McLeish, J., Redshaw, M., 2019. Maternity experiences of mothers with multiple disadvantages in England: a qualitative study. Women Birth 32 (2), 178–184.

Murray, L., Windsor, C., Parker, E., Tewfik, O., 2010. The experiences of African women giving birth in Brisbane, Australia. Health Care Women Int. 31 (5), 458–472.

Ndirangu, E.W., Evans, C., 2009. Experiences of African immigrant women living with HIV in the UK: implications for health professionals. J Immigr Minor Health. 11 (2), 108–114.

Nellums, L.B., Rustage, K., Hargreaves, S., Friedland, J., Miller, A., Hiam, L., 2018. Access to Healthcare for People Seeking and Refused Asylum in Great Britain: A Review of Evidence. Equality and Human Rights Commission.

National Institute for Health and Care Excellence, 2016. Diversity, equality and language. Antenatal and postnatal mental health. Available at: https://www.nice.org.uk/guidance/qs115/chapter/Diversity-equality-and-language.

National Maternity Review, 2016. Better Births: improving outcomes of maternity services in England. NHS England. Available at: https://www.england.nhs.uk/wp-content/uploads/2016/02/national-maternity-review-report.pdf.

Niner, S., Kokanovic, R., Cuthbert, D., 2013. Displaced mothers: birth and resettlement, gratitude and complaint. Med. Anthropol. 32 (6), 535–551.

O'Mahony, J.M., Donnelly, T.T., 2007. The influence of culture on immigrant women's mental health care experiences from the perspectives of health care providers. Issues Ment. Health Nurs. 28 (5), 453–471.

Origlia Ikhilor, P., Hasenberg, G., Kurth, E., Asefaw, F., Pehlke-Milde, J., Cignacco, E., 2019. Communication barriers in maternity care of allophone migrants: experiences of women, healthcare professionals, and intercultural interpreters. J. Adv. Nurs. 75 (10), 2200–2210.

Owens, C., Dandy, J., Hancock, P., 2016. Perceptions of pregnancy experiences when using a community-based antenatal service: a qualitative study of refugee and migrant women in Perth, Western Australia. Women Birth 29 (2), 128–137.

Pangas, J., Ogunsiji, O., Elmir, R., Raman, S., Liamputtong, P., Burns, E., et al., 2019. Refugee women's experiences negotiating motherhood and maternity care in a new country: a meta-ethnographic review. Int. J. Nurs. Stud. 90, 31–45.

Phelan, J.C., Lucas, J.W., Ridgeway, C.L., Taylor, C.J., 2014. Stigma, status, and population health. Soc. Sci. Med. 103, 15–23.

Phillimore, J., 2015. Delivering maternity services in an era of superdiversity: the challenges of novelty and newness. Ethn. Racial Stud. 38 (4), 568–582.

Public Health England, 2020. Beyond the data: understanding the impact of Covid-19 on BAME communities. Available at: https://www.gov.uk/government/publications/covid-19-understanding-the-impact-on-bame-communities.

Purnell, L.D., Paulanka, B.J., 1998. Transcultural Health Care: A Culturally Competent Approach. F.A. Davis, Philadelphia.

Puthussery, S., 2016. Perinatal outcomes among migrant mothers in the United Kingdom: is it a matter of biology, behaviour, policy, social determinants or access to health care? Best Pract. Res. Clin. Obstet. Gynaecol. 32, 39–49.

Randall, V., 2019. Race, racism and the law. https://racism.org

Rayment-Jones, H., Harris, J., Harden, A., Khan, Z., Sandall, J., 2019. How do women with social risk factors experience United Kingdom maternity care? A realist synthesis. Birth 46 (3), 461–474.

Razai, M.S., Kankam, H.K., Majeed, A., Esmail, A., Williams, D.R., 2021. Mitigating ethnic disparities in covid-19 and beyond. BMJ 372, m4921.

RCM, 2018. Midwifery Continuity of Carer Model. https://www.rcm.org.uk/media/2946/midwifery-continuity-of-carer-mcoc.pdf#:~:text=the%20RCM%20is%20continuity%20across%20the%20whole%20continuum%3A,midwifery%20continuity%20model%20works%20within%20and%20alongside%20the

Rivenbark, J.G., Ichou, M., 2020. Discrimination in healthcare as a barrier to care: experiences of socially disadvantaged populations in France from a nationally representative survey. BMC Public Health 20 (1), 1–10.

Rosenthal, L., Overstreet, N.M., Woods-Giscombe, C.L., Lewis, T., 2016. Addressing Health Disparities Faced by Black and Latina Women: Research Participation, Health Risks, Health Care Utilization. in Annals of Behavioral Medicine, 50. Journals dept, 2001 Evans RD, Cary, NC, US: Oxford University Press Inc., S45–S45.

Russo, A., Lewis, B., Joyce, A., Crockett, B., Luchters, S., 2015. A qualitative exploration of the emotional wellbeing and support needs of new mothers from Afghanistan living in Melbourne, Australia. BMC Pregnancy Childbirth 15 (1), 1–13.

Sartori, P., 2010. Spirituality 1: should spiritual and religious beliefs be part of patient care? Nurs. Times 106 (28), 14–17.

Schyve, P.M., 2007. Language differences as a barrier to quality and safety in health care: the Joint Commission perspective. J. Gen. Intern. Med. 22 (2), 360–361.

Shafiei, T., Small, R., McLachlan, H., 2012. Women's views and experiences of maternity care: a study of immigrant Afghan women in Melbourne, Australia. Midwifery 28 (2), 198–203.

Shieh, C., Mays, R., McDaniel, A., Yu, J., 2009. Health literacy and its association with the use of information sources and with barriers to information seeking in clinic-based pregnant women. Health Care Women Int 30 (11), 971–988.

Singleton, K., Krause, E., 2009. Understanding cultural and linguistic barriers to health literacy. The Online Journal of Issues in Nursing 14 (3) Available at: https://ojin.nursingworld.org/MainMenuCategories/ANAMarketplace/ANAPeriodicals/OJIN/TableofContents/Vol142009/No3Sept09/Cultural-and-Linguistic-Barriers-.aspx

Sørensen, K., Van den Broucke, S., Fullam, J., Doyle, G., Pelikan, J., Slonska, Z., Brand, H., 2012. Health literacy and public health: a systematic review and integration of definitions and models. BMC Public Health 12 (1), 1–13.

Spencer, S.J., Logel, C., Davies, P.G., 2016. Stereotype threat. Ann. Rev. Psychol. 67, 415–437.

Stapleton, H., Murphy, R., Correa-Velez, I., Steel, M., Kildea, S., 2013. Women from refugee backgrounds and their experiences of attending a specialist antenatal clinic. Narratives from an Australian setting. Women Birth 26 (4), 260–266.

Stewart, M., Dennis, C.L., Kariwo, M., Kushner, K.E., Letourneau, N., Makumbe, K., et al., 2015. Challenges faced by refugee new parents from Africa in Canada. J. Immigr. Minor. Health 17 (4), 1146–1156.

Sudbury, H., Robinson, A., 2016. Barriers to sexual and reproductive health care for refugee and asylum-seeking women. Br. J. Midwifery 24 (4), 275–281.

Tobin, C.L., Murphy-Lawless, J., 2014. Irish midwives' experiences of providing maternity care to non-Irish women seeking asylum. International Journal of Women's Health 6, 159.

Truong, M., Paradies, Y., Priest, N., 2014. Interventions to improve cultural competency in healthcare: a systematic review of reviews. BMC Health Serv. Res. 14 (1), 1–17.

Wheeler, E., 1998. Mental illness and social stigma: experiences in a Pakistani community in the UK. J. Gend Dev. 6 (1), 37–43.

Williams, D.R., Mohammed, S.A., 2013. Racism and health II: a needed research agenda for effective interventions. Am. Behav. Sci. 57 (8), 1200–1226.

Wilson, R., Sanders, M., Dumper, H., 2007. Sexual Health, Asylum Seekers and Refugees: a Handbook for People Working with Refugees and Asylum Seekers in England. Family Planning Association, London.

Wojnar, D.M., 2015. Perinatal experiences of Somali couples in the United States. J. Obstet. Gynecol. Neonatal Nurs. 44 (3), 358–369.

World Health Organization, 2003. Working with Individuals, Families and Communities to Improve Maternal and Newborn Health (No. WHO/FCH/RHR/03.11). World Health Organization, Geneva.

World Health Organization, 2006. Quality of Care: a Process for Making Strategic Choices in Health Systems. World Health Organization. Available at: https://www.who.int/management/quality/assurance/QualityCare_B.Def.pdf.

World Health Organization, 2014. The prevention and elimination of disrespect and abuse during facility-based childbirth. Available at: http://apps.who.int/iris/bitstream/handle/10665/134588/WHO_RHR_14.23_eng.pdf?sequence=1.

World Health Organization, 2015. Fact sheet No 351: Family planning/contraception. Available at: www.who.int/mediacentre/factsheets/fs351/en.

World Health Organization, 2021. Developing quality standards for maternal and newborn care. Available at: https://www.who.int/maternal_child_adolescent/topics/quality-of-care/en/.

Ethical Issues in Transcultural Care

This chapter will begin with a discussion on the meaning of ethics and provide an overview of the main bioethical principles of respect for autonomy, beneficence, non-maleficence and justice. You will also examine the issues of privacy, confidentiality, veracity and fidelity in relation to clinical midwifery practice and how these elements can be facilitated when providing midwifery care. The midwife's role in ensuring good ethical practice and considering alternatives if there is conflict between the woman's culture and the professional/organisational culture will be included. This chapter ends with the organisational factors that affect good ethical practice and discusses the importance of acknowledging these issues at individual and organisational levels.

Ethical Practice

WHAT IS ETHICS

Ethics is a broad term that covers the study of the nature of morals and specific moral choices (Varkey, 2021). It is determining what is right or wrong. The word 'ethics' means character and is derived from the Greek word 'ethos'. In healthcare, ethics play an important role in ensuring that individuals are treated well and with consideration. Another way of understanding ethics is that these are moral principles that control how a person behaves, and every person has their own set of personal ethics and morals. The terms 'ethics' and 'morals' are used interchangeably, but ethics are essentially influenced by external forces, such as workplace policies and professional codes, whereas morals are personally driven. Some moral norms for proper conduct are common to all humans as they transcend cultures, regions, religions and constitute common morality such as not to kill or cause harm, not to steal, not to punish the innocent, to be truthful and to obey the law (Varkey, 2021).

BIOETHICS

The application of ethics to healthcare settings is known as bioethics. The value of bioethics in healthcare is a shared understanding and knowledge between healthcare professionals about how healthcare should be conducted. Bioethics is not only helpful in providing a guideline for health professionals and clinical decision-making but is valuable for policy development and legislation (Taj and Khan, 2018). Ethics within midwifery practice is important because you must recognise healthcare dilemmas and make sound judgements and decisions based on your values, while keeping within the laws that govern them (Haddad and Geiger, 2018). You should always be consciously aware of the decisions and judgements you make daily, and how you react has an enormous impact on a woman's rights. Ogston-Tuck (2014) states that a healthcare professional needs to be aware of the existence of a moral or ethical situation before they can be ethical. Therefore, the midwife needs a basic understanding of what constitutes a moral or ethical incident before she can undertake appropriate action or behaviour.

PRINCIPLISM

Principlism is an ethical problem–solving method outlined by Beauchamp and Childress (2009), guiding professionals in practising ethically, ensuring that the rights of childbearing women are respected with the overriding principle of care based on the obligation to see those rights maintained. You should practice the basic tenets of principlism, which is guided by professional governance. The Nursing and Midwifery Council (NMC, 2018) Code reflects these principles of putting patients and service users first by promoting professionalism, trust, safety and effective care. You have a statutory obligation to adhere to the NMC Code. Consideration of women's cultural and diverse needs is referred to in the Code (Table 6.1, NMC, 2018).

The International Code of Ethics from the International Confederation of Midwives (ICM) addresses the midwife's mandate to uphold professional responsibilities and duties and to work to ensure the integrity of the profession of midwifery (ICM, 2018). Therefore, you should have a good understanding of ethical principles and their relevance to everyday practice.

The core of healthcare ethics is four bioethical principles: respect for autonomy, nonmaleficence beneficence and justice (Beauchamp, 2007) (Fig. 6.1). There are also the behavioural norms of veracity, privacy, confidentiality and fidelity. These moral and behavioural norms share common elements mainly in autonomy, beneficence and nonmaleficence. To practice ethically requires you to have awareness and sensitivity for the woman as an individual, including her cultural values and beliefs (Hoop et al., 2008). A person can achieve cultural competency by adhering to ethical principles.

TABLE 6.1 ■ Elements Addressing Cultural Diversity in the NMC Code

Prioritise people	Women should be treated with kindness, respect and compassion
	Avoid making assumptions and recognise diversity and individual choice
	Respect and uphold human rights
	Act as an advocate for the vulnerable and challenge poor and discriminatory attitudes
	Get properly informed consent
	Respect the woman's right to privacy and confidentiality
Practice effectively	Communicate with women clearly
	Take reasonable steps to meet the woman's language needs and consider cultural sensitivities to better understand the woman's personal and health needs
Preserve safety	Put right the situation if a woman has suffered harm or if an incident has happened which has caused her harm
	Take all reasonable steps to protect women who are vulnerable or at risk from harm, neglect or abuse
Promote pro-fessionalism	Act with honesty and integrity at all times. Do not express your personal beliefs (including political, religious or moral beliefs) to people in an inappropriate way

Adapted from NMC, 2018. The code: professional standards of practice and behaviour for nurses and midwives. https://www.nmc.org.uk/standards/code/read-the-code-online/.

Moral Principles

BENEFICENCE

In short, beneficence means 'to do good'. Beneficence is the duty of a midwife to always act for the benefit of the woman, her baby and her family. To do this, you must prevent harm, avoid situations that may cause harm and consistently seek to benefit the woman. It is natural to think that all healthcare professionals would practice beneficence; however, the case is that any intervention or treatment can cause harm. Therefore, you must develop and maintain knowledge and skills in the latest evidence-based midwifery practice to reduce harm. This stance is also required to ensure that women are offered the best available and appropriate midwifery care. The issue with beneficence

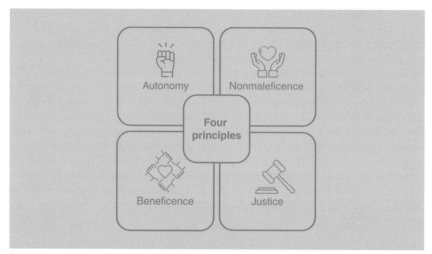

Fig. 6.1 The four principles of healthcare ethics. (Modified from https://clipboardhealth.com/how-the-4-principles-of-health-care-ethics-improve-patient-care.)

is determining what 'good' means to the woman. You should be cognisant that what is appropriate for one woman may not be so for another.

NONMALEFICENCE

Nonmaleficence is simply acting in a way so as not to harm women. To be precise, nonmaleficence means to 'do no harm'. In other words, the midwife must act so as not to intervene or advise treatments that will not be the best outcome for the woman. The four factors to consider in nonmaleficence are that any act should not be wrong, every act should have a positive benefit, a good effect should not come about due to a wrong action and any good outcomes should always outweigh harmful consequences (Drysdale, 2020). Therefore, you have a choice of doing nothing about a problem or to do something about a problem rather than risk causing harm.

RESPECT FOR AUTONOMY

Respect for autonomy refers to the fact that all individuals should have the power to make rational decisions and moral choices and be allowed to exercise a capacity for self-determination (Varkey, 2021). A woman should have the right to maintain control of her body during pregnancy. Practising autonomy prevents you from the potential of persuading a woman to undertake a specific intervention or treatment. The woman should be allowed to make decisions about her pregnancy rather than be told what to do. As already stated, care delivered to a woman should be evidence-based. This also ensures that you are not providing care based on your own beliefs and values. If a midwife recognises that every woman has the right to decide what happens to her body and her baby, this means she is respected as an individual and that her choices are a result of personal values and beliefs.

JUSTICE

Justice is the duty to treat women fairly and equally. This involves fairness in all decisions made about a woman and assessing the advantages and disadvantages of any care or treatment provided.

You have a professional obligation to provide justice to all women. Alperovitch et al. (2009) state there are two elements of the principle of justice, namely, equality and equity. Equality, for example, means offering the same access and opportunities to healthcare and services to all women, whilst equity recognises that each woman has different circumstances and healthcare should be allocated to achieve an equal outcome for everyone. Several factors may influence justice and a woman's rights during pregnancy, for example, age, place of residence, social status, ethnic background and culture.

Gillon (1994) emphasises that justice is more than mere equality in that people can be treated unjustly even if they are treated equally. With reference to Aristotle, Gillon (2003) argues that it is important to treat equals equally and unequal's unequally in proportion to the morally relevant inequalities. Therefore, you should assess the needs of each woman before any care and treatment and adjust services and care to ensure equity.

The promotion of autonomy for all women is an application of the ethical principle of justice. When women are treated fairly and equally, this leads to supporting their rights to decide for themselves.

While justice usually has been used regarding a standard of rightness, fairness often has been used with regard to an ability to judge without reference to one's feelings or interests. Fairness has also been used to refer to the ability to make judgements that are not overly general but concrete and specific to a particular case (Velasquez et al., 2014). When individuals have different views over what they believe should be given, or when decisions must be made about how benefits should be distributed among a group of people, questions of justice or fairness inevitably arise (Velasquez et al., 2014).

MORAL UNIVERSALISM AND ABSOLUTISM

Moral universalism is a concept that believes that ethics can be applied universally regardless of culture, race, religion, sexual orientation or nationality. Therefore, ethics is said to transcend cultures. The universal approach is said to simplify the decision-making process as the ethical choice has essentially been predetermined. Hence, reflection and debate are not necessary. The universal approach is typically used in cross-cultural situations, but it may also be used in any situation where one person behaves outside of the culturally accepted norm.

Moral absolutism is the idea that if something is not right in one place or for one person, then it is not right for anyone in any context. Moral absolutism is not the same as universalism which states that what is right or wrong is independent of custom or opinion but not necessarily that what is right or wrong is independent of context or consequences. In other words, in universalism, there is some allowance for immoral behaviour depending on the situation or outcomes. However, in midwifery practice, the nature of the midwife/woman relationship means that certain moral absolutes will always apply, such as not being abusive or disrespectful to a woman.

CULTURAL RELATIVISM

Cultural relativism proposes that different cultures have different codes of conduct and moral standards (Yeung, 2017). This is an important concept, as it suggests that there is no universal code to judge others. Cultural relativism challenges the belief in objectivity and universality of moral truths; in effect, there is no universal truth in ethics and only cultural codes (Table 6.2). For example, if a woman from a non-Western culture is being cared for, then Western values may be inappropriate. Hence, you should understand a woman's culture on its terms and not judge her morals or values. Cultural relativism suggests that no one culture is more superior to another based on morality. In addition, any view of ethical behaviour may be subjective to each woman in a particular culture.

TABLE 6.2 ■ **Examples of Cultural Relativism**

Religious traditions – Baptism, Communion	Rules on dress and nudity
Role of children	Rules on sexuality
Issues of privacy	Rules on gender equality

When discussing human rights, the term 'cultural relativism' creates confusion because it refers to a view that all cultures are equal and secondary to universal values when examining cultural norms (Reichert, 2015). This leads to the stance that external values are inferior to that of the local culture, which can raise dilemmas. For example, if local cultures allow female genital mutilation (FGM), then the international consensus that FGM is a barbaric practice is irrelevant (Reichert, 2011). Hence, there is an argument that cultural relativism is an outdated concept. Cultural relativism shapes what an individual would consider to be appealing or abhorrent. A person's view may vary not just in terms of national cultures but within large societies and cultures and subcultures organised by class, race, sexuality, region, religion and ethnicity (Cole, 2020).

Cultural relativism is an important concept to consider in midwifery, as it provides a worldview and understanding of other cultures.

CULTURAL RELATIVISM VERSUS MORAL UNIVERSALISM

Cultural relativism has several positives. One is that an explanation is provided for why individuals have different values and accommodation of cultural expression. In addition, cultural relativism prevents one culture from becoming dominant over another. However, one negative of cultural relativism is that it is impossible to have one moral truth, as there are different value systems. Difficulties arise as there is the existence of many views which are not all equally true. This difficulty is overcome by universalism (Fig. 6.2), where there is a fixed moral code. The United National Declaration of Human Rights states a set of absolutes that apply to all people regardless of country. Supporters of universality believe that the human rights guaranteed in international treaties and conventions should be applied in all countries, and that they must prevail even when they conflict with established cultural or religious practices (Musalo, 2015).

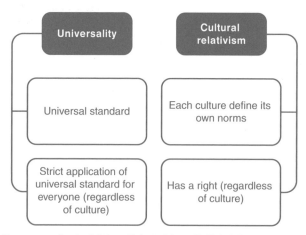

Fig. 6.2 Universality versus cultural relativism. (Adapted from IB Global Politics, 2021. Cultural Relativism and Universal Human Rights. https://sites.google.com/a/isb.be/isbglobalpolitics/unit-human-rights/cultural-relativism-and-universal-human-rights.)

Donnelly (1984) provides the following perspectives of cultural relativism and universal human rights.

The Universal Declaration of Human Rights is an approach that views human rights as prima facie (accepted as correct until proven otherwise) universal, but recognises culture as a limited source of exceptions and multiple interpretations.

Cultural relativism gives too much potential for abuse, with those in power able to dictate what determines 'culture' to hide abuses of power.

Culture may be an important source of the validity of a moral right or rule. In other words, there is a weak presumption of universality, but the relativity of human nature, communities and rights serves as a check on potential excesses of universalism.

There is near universal international agreement, at least in theory, although often not in practice, that certain things simply cannot legitimately be done to human beings- regardless of the difficulties in specifying those things. Failure to act or even speak out against the grossest affronts to human dignity overseas on the grounds of cultural relativism would be widely - and I believe correctly - perceived as moral cowardice.

Cultural relativism states that values are defined by local culture as opposed to global ideology. Cultural relativists also argue that human rights were developed by Western countries and are based on Western morality. Therefore, they should not be imposed on non-Western societies that have different histories, cultures and levels of development. In response, universalists argue that ideals like liberty and security belong to every human being. There is criticism of cultural relativist arguments, which is seen as an attempt to justify the oppression of minorities or defend harmful cultural practices.

Moral absolutism also attracts criticism as circumstances of behaviour are not taken into consideration. For example, cultural practices such as intermarriage and childbearing rituals may be deemed immoral in moral absolutism regardless of context. Hence, it can seem that to apply moral universalism or absolutism to some cultural behaviour may be inappropriate. However, some researchers have argued that it is possible to adopt a cultural relativist stance without abandoning a commitment to the idea of universal standards or human rights (Li, 2007).

Due to the debate between cultural relativism and universalism, it may be challenging to determine when each term applies in any situation. IB Global Politics (2021) have devised some analytical tests to evaluate claims of cultural relativism and universalism (Table 6.3).

Practice Point

The concepts of universalism, moral absolutism and cultural relativism are relevant in midwifery practice. You are governed by the NMC Code of conduct which can be used as a tool to ensure the care provided to women is ethical. The NMC Code can be used as a guide for practice that adheres to universalism and moral absolutism. However, challenges may arise when you are faced with a moral situation that has tenets of cultural relativism requiring careful consideration of the woman's wishes and, more importantly, her human rights.

Culture and Moral Principles
CULTURAL COMPETENCE AND ETHICAL DECISION-MAKING

Applications of ethical principles in cultural settings vary more often from one cultural perspective to another because of the different understanding and practices of what is good

TABLE 6.3 ■ Analytical Tests

• Cultural relativism test	• The practice should be defensible within the basic value framework of the society or culture. Practices that do not stand up to such evaluations can in no sense be defended on cultural terms
• Universalism test	• The presumption is that human rights can be applied universally. Human rights are universal unless proven otherwise by a particular cultural argument.
• Validity test	• Is the action a principled action or a self-interested action?
• Avoidance of harm test	• Harm is considered to have taken place when there is death, pain, disability, loss of freedom or pleasure that results from an act by one human upon another
	• The notion of harm done to individuals or groups can be used to explore the ground between universal rights and cultural relativism. When reasonable persons from different cultural backgrounds agree that certain institutions or cultural practices cause harm, then the moral neutrality of cultural relativism is suspended

Adapted from IB Global Politics, 2021. Cultural relativism and universal human rights. https://sites.google.com/a/isb.be/isbglobalpolitics/unit-human-rights/cultural-relativism-and-universal-human-rights.

(Chukwuneke et al., 2014). Cultural competence and ethical decision-making are inseparable in clinical practice (Louw, 2016). You need to utilise both skills when caring for women. You should appreciate that moral principles are not prioritised in the same way across the globe and that respect for autonomy does not conflict necessarily with acceptance of other cultures' beliefs about the importance of community (e.g., autonomy [self-rule] would allow an individual to accept their 'role' within a family willingly) (Minkoff, 2014). Some cultural and religious obligations may be seen as morally obligatory for members of those cultures or religions but not a moral obligation for others (Gillon, 2003). A midwife who is culturally competent and culturally safe has the ability to make ethical decisions regarding any woman's care regardless of her culture. The skill of being culturally sensitive supports the skill of empathy and understanding required in ethical decision-making.

CULTURE, BENEFICENCE AND NONMALEFICENCE

Beneficence and nonmaleficence are based on values shared by people from many other cultures. However, the concept of 'doing good' in Western society may have more relevance than in a non-Western society as there is also a deeply held belief in the changeability of the future and the importance of acting rather than simply being (Hoop et al., 2008). Beneficence and nonmaleficence in cultural settings vary more often from one cultural perspective to the other because of the different understanding and practices of 'what is good' (Chukwuneke et al., 2014). Beneficence has arisen in Western medicine from the traditional paternalistic approach adopted in doctor-patient relationships. In non-Western medicine, similar ethical principles are also practised. Aksoy and Tenik (2002) state the existence of the four principles in the Islamic tradition with a clear emphasis on the principle of beneficence. In China, medical ethics also has a great emphasis on beneficence in that Chinese medicine is considered 'a humane art, and a physician must be loving to treat the sick and heal the injured' (Kao, 2002). Causing harm means different things to African societies; for example, the use of stem cells or embryo for any form of clinical or research work is regarded as murder in most African societies; the Western world, however, may have no issues with this due to the benefits to society (Chukwuneke et al., 2014).

AUTONOMY IN DIFFERENT CULTURES

Culture plays a key role by setting boundaries for the appropriate level of autonomy for individuals within a society (Chirkov, 2017). In societies that have strong social structures that rigidly define the roles of men and women encoded in religious, tribal and social traditions, some constraints may define the circumstances under which women have or do not have the autonomy to make decisions regarding their own health (Osamor and Grady, 2016). Respect for autonomy is more clearly tied to Western cultural values, and particularly the value placed on human beings as individuals rather than members of a group (Kitchener, 2000). The idea of individualistic autonomy may be ill-suited to other cultures. The importance of social relationships to an individual's social relationships should be considered. Relational autonomy, which highlights the context in which all individuals exist, acknowledges the emotional aspects of being autonomous. Relational autonomy in different cultures is particularly relevant to reproductive health, which may directly impact family members. Individuals may be ill-equipped to deal with these kinds of decisions in an individualistic, autonomous manner (Osamor and Grady, 2016).

There may be particularly little freedom of choice for women in India, the Middle East, and North Africa. Studies from South Asia (Senarath and Gunawardena, 2009) reported that women's autonomy and decision to seek healthcare were allocated as determined by social and cultural factors. The African ethical framework focuses on the community good rather than the individual, which is different from Western ethics that emphasises the autonomy, freedom and moral inclination of the individual (Chukwuneke et al., 2014). Many cultures practice patrilocality, in which a married couple lives near or with the husband's parents; when a woman gets married, she essentially ceases to be a member of her birth family and joins her husband's family (Jayachandran, 2015). Therefore, the individual autonomy of the woman becomes aligned to the family. Co-residence of adult sons and elderly parents is much more common in Asia, the Middle East and North Africa than in Europe, sub-Saharan Africa and the Americas (Ebenstein, 2014). In Chinese cultures, the head of the family is the one who makes decisions on behalf of his family members; there may be discussion of the issues with the family members, but the final decision rests with the head of the family (Tai and Lin, 2001; Tai and Tsai, 2003).

Understanding the difference between a woman's autonomy and social support is important. For example, when a woman makes a joint decision with a husband/partner or others, you may interpret this as indicating lower autonomy for the woman; however, making a decision alone may represent simply lack of support from a husband/partner who would rather not be involved (Carlson et al., 2015). As a woman is most likely to be embedded in her social context, her decisions often take into account consideration for others in her household and community, and decisions may not be, or appear not to be, fully autonomous (Osamor and Grady, 2016).

It is important for you to understand how culturally shaped views of autonomy impact the role of the woman in the family. Respecting autonomy within other cultures involves giving preference to other ethical values such as fidelity and family connections and community over individual decision-making (Segal and Hodges, 2012). Although midwives have guidelines for their interaction with the women based on clear principles, they should still adapt those principles to the woman's culture (Di Mattia, 2008).

Practice Point

It is important to recognise that cultural beliefs and values or religion impact considerably on the meaning of the concepts of autonomy, beneficence, nonmaleficence and justice. The emphasis should be on you recognising that these ethical principles are valued differently in other cultures.

Behavioural Norms

PRIVACY

Privacy is a basic human right and is universally recognised. It is used as an umbrella term that covers many concepts such as confidentiality, security and secrecy. Conceptualisation of privacy according to Finn et al. (2013) may be necessary to maintain a fluidity that enables new dimensions of privacy to be identified, understood and addressed. Seven types of privacy discussed by Finn et al. (2013) are:

- **Privacy of the person** – the right to body functions and characteristics being kept private
- **Privacy of behaviour and action** – includes sexual preferences, political activities and cultural/religious practices
- **Privacy of communication** – any verbal communication but also email, telephone and recordings
- **Privacy of data and image** – individual's data is not automatically available to other organisations
- **Privacy of thoughts and feelings** – people have the right not to share thoughts or feelings or have them revealed
- **Privacy of location and space** – right to solitude and right to privacy in spaces
- **Privacy of association** – right to associate with others; for example, politically, for worship, **privacy of association also connects to groupings or profiles over which we have no control – for example, DNA testing can reveal that we are members of a particular ethnic group or a particular family**

Privacy is also conceptualised as a multi-dimensional construct consisting of four theoretically independent dimensions: social, informational, physical and psychological (Fig. 6.3) (Leino-Kilpi, 2000; Serenko and Fan, 2013). Physical privacy is the degree to which one is physically accessible to others and is related to the concepts of personal space and territoriality, which, as discussed in a previous chapter, can be culturally derived (Leino-Kilpi et al., 2001). Psychological privacy concerns the ability of a person to control cognitive and affective thoughts, to form values and the right to determine with whom and under what circumstances they will share thoughts or reveal intimate information (Burgoon, 1982). Social privacy is an individual's ability to control how they socially interact with other people and has strong cultural meanings. In addition, social privacy entails being free from actual interaction with others and any perceived pressures on one's own course of action (Burgoon, 1982).

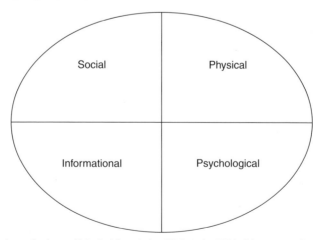

Fig. 6.3 Dimensions of privacy. (Adapted from Leino-Kilpi et al., 2001. Privacy: a review of the literature. Int. J. Nurs. Stud. 38 (6), 663–671.)

Informational privacy relates to an individual's right to determine how, when and to what extent information about the self will be released to another person. Informational privacy is a key component of the overall privacy perceptions of healthcare users, followed by physical privacy. Privacy has a strong effect on trust, which in turn affects the level of commitment, intentions to use the provider's services in the future, and engagement in positive word-of-mouth (Serenko and Fan, 2013).

Autonomy has been related to privacy as it allows self-determining and control on who can access a person. Personal privacy can be defined as preventing access to physical space as well as access to information. In addition, privacy includes personal choices such as cultural and religious affiliations (decisional privacy) and personal relationships with family members and other close persons (associational privacy).

Decisional privacy offers individuals the freedom to act and make important decisions about how they live without unjustifiable interference from other individuals (Dimopoulos, 2021). It is argued that decisional privacy is valued as a condition that enables individual autonomy.

CONFIDENTIALITY

Confidentiality can be defined as an 'ethical principle in which information about an individual is made accessible only to those who require it' (Tiran, 2012). Confidentiality is also about you respecting a woman's wishes about how her personal details are shared with others. The main difference between confidentiality and privacy is that privacy can be 'invaded', while confidentiality is 'breached' (Francis, 2008). There are several regulations that a midwife should adhere to regarding confidentiality. The Human Rights Act (1998) gives every woman the right to have the privacy of her family respected. The NMC (2018) states that every person has a right to confidentiality, and you must ensure each person in your care receives it.

The National Health Service (NHS) Confidentiality Code of Practice (2003) outlines four primary requirements that must be met to provide women with a confidential service:

- Protect women's information.
- Inform women of how their information is used.
- Allow women to decide whether their information can be shared.
- Look for improved ways to protect, inform and provide choices to women.

Apart from confidentiality being a woman's right, a breach of confidentiality can lead to a breakdown of trust. Therefore, you must take all steps to avoid this occurrence.

VERACITY (TRUTH-TELLING)

The principle of veracity (truth-telling) requires healthcare personnel to provide comprehensive, accurate and objective information in a manner that helps patients understand the information (Sorrell, 2017). There can be a conflict between autonomy and beneficence, which can impact truth-telling in some cultures. Telling the woman the truth ensures that the woman receives the correct information that she can use to make the correct choice. Explaining the truth to the woman is a highly complex process, and the midwife's experience is very important; a midwife who has developed good communication skills can give the amount of information that the woman wants and when she is ready (Amer, 2019). Truth-telling promotes trust and respect, and it also prevents harm, as women who are uninformed about their situation may fail to access midwifery care when they should.

FIDELITY

Fidelity is the principle concerned with building trusting relationships between midwives and women. Beauchamp and Childress (2013) believe that fidelity is best understood when related to the ethical principles of autonomy and justice. When caring for a woman, you have an obligation to protect each woman, as far as possible, from any harm. Fidelity means that you must be faithful to the promises you make as a professional to provide competent, quality care to women. Fidelity is also said to govern the other ethical principles and requires treating all women with respect. This is not always easy, especially if the woman is disrespectful or discourteous. Midwives should ensure that any negative feelings they might have about caring for any woman should be put aside and provide the standard of care required.

Culture and Behavioural Norms

PRIVACY AND CULTURE

Privacy is culturally defined and is influenced by cultural values and beliefs (Low et al., 2007). Culture has an impact on how people try to maintain their privacy. Privacy which is seen as a fundamental principle in individuals from Western cultures encompassing an individual's an freedom, personal identity, private space and interactions with other people (Beauchamp and Childress, 2013). However, privacy in other cultures can denote other factors of which the midwife should be aware of. For example, physical privacy may be a matter of cultural sensitivity, personal dignity and shyness. Privacy could also be about access to the woman (her body, her choices and certain types of information about her) (Estroff and Walker, 2012). A woman maintaining privacy is seen to show respect for religion, culture and community and being respected in return. For example, respect for religion may refer to Islam and its rules on what should be kept private, such as women using veils (Eklöf et al., 2015). In Judaism, respect for religion also results in women covering the head and not exposing their hair. The woman will determine what type of privacy is important to her, and this will vary between women and be influenced by culture, religion and socioeconomic factors.

Eklof et al. (2015), in a study of migrant African women, suggested that privacy can be defined by content or importance. The content and significance of privacy could also be divided into sub-themes (Fig. 6.4) (Eklöf et al., 2015).

Visual privacy refers to the body, who should see it and is of great importance in many cultures. As discussed in the previous chapter, in some cultures, only another female should see a woman's body, and only the woman's husband may view her body. In cultures where clothing is used to protect a woman's visual privacy, this is particularly important. Justification for revealing the body to a different gender would usually be for health reasons. However, you would need to clarify the reason for invading a woman's visual privacy; otherwise, it may be seen as a sign of disrespect.

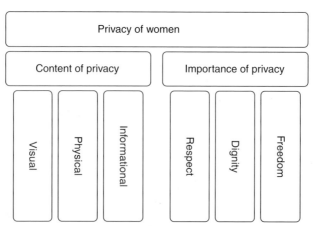

Fig. 6.4 Content of privacy versus importance of privacy. (Adapted from Eklöf et al., 2016. Somali asylum seekers' perceptions of privacy in healthcare. Nurs Ethics. 23 (5), 535–546.)

Physical privacy refers to touch; again in some cultures, for example, African and Asian women and religions such as Islam and Judaism, touch should only be from family members and healthcare professionals of the same gender (Eklöf et al., 2015; Selekman and Zavadivker, 2021). In some cases, even touch from a healthcare professional of the same gender would be seen as disrespectful unless the justification is clear.

Informational privacy wishes vary according to different cultures; the woman may not want to share information with others, including family members or healthcare professionals and interpreters. Culturally, some topics are taboo topics such as sexual and mental health, which should not be discussed outside the family. Also, such information should only be discussed with the same gender; this is pertinent to sexual health matters. In some communities, women may be concerned about the intimacies of a small community where the interpreter speaks the same language and comes from the same community. The woman may fear the sharing of personal information, which may be spread by gossip. Hence, some women may decline an interpreter.

Privacy is also seen to be a way of protecting dignity. Dignity refers not only to the dignity of an individual but also the dignity of the community. While being respected by the community refers to something conveyed from the community to the individual, dignity is also described as being something conveyed from the individual to the community.

Freedom refers to the woman's individual choice to show, talk or share personal things with others. Even if it is seen as a woman's freedom, it is guided by religion and culture (Eklöf et al., 2015). However, the level of freedom is seen to be strongly related to the society the woman lives in.

Practice Point

You may face the challenge of understanding how privacy differs in women from other cultures. The midwife can easily achieve some aspects of privacy, such as ensuring the woman's wishes to keep her body covered. Other aspects require more facilitation but should be recognised as equally important to the woman and therefore accommodated if possible.

CONFIDENTIALLY AND CULTURE

When applied to confidentiality, beneficence and nonmaleficence result in protecting the woman's personal information and possible breach of confidentiality due to the need to minimise the risk of harm. A woman's right to confidentiality lies in her right to autonomy. You should not disclose information given by a woman to another party, except for sharing necessary health information for the woman's care. In particular, discipline should be exercised in sharing information with the woman's family.

Your role as a midwife involves caring for the woman holistically; this involves retrieving pertinent information from the woman to provide the best care. To do this, you need to form a relationship with the woman and create trust. Another crucial factor is that you need to encourage the woman to share information so that the most appropriate advice can be provided.

There are circumstances where you may break confidentiality if it is done to protect the woman's best interest or the interests of the public. There are several exceptions which include sharing cultural/religious practices that are harmful, for example, the practice of FGM. There has been a mandatory requirement since 31 October 2015 for health professionals to report to the police all cases of FGM in girls under 18 and record any cases of FGM in women over 18 (NHS, England, 2020). However, the benefits of mandatory data submission do not automatically outweigh the potential harm to the woman/midwife relationship and public trust. There is a concern that without assurance of confidentiality, women who have had FGM may avoid revealing their condition (Naftalin and Bewley, 2015); this may also apply to other cultural practices.

In the first instance, in your practice you may retrieve information from the woman of any cultural practices that she performs or intends to perform in pregnancy. A dilemma you may face is the need to report cultural practices that the woman adheres to during pregnancy that are deemed to be harmful. This could vary from unsafe feeding practices of the neonate to the use of unprescribed medicines or herbs, for example. Breaches of confidentiality, then, can have doubly negative consequences—both harm to the woman (by making the formerly private information public) and damage to her trust in the mother/midwife relationship, which is crucial for managing the pregnancy (Estroff and Walker, 2012).

VERACITY AND CULTURE

In some cultures, family members may request that the truth be withheld, usually to prevent what is perceived as possible harm to their loved one. Systematic reviews suggest collusion (defined as a cultural practice in which family members request withholding information from the patient) is common in regions where families, rather than individual patients, are considered the central element of healthcare decision-making (Yeung, 2017). A midwife should be open to such diverse perspectives, allowing rapport building and working with families collaboratively. If the midwife disregards cultural values, this may damage the mother/midwife relationship and harm the quality of care.

Midwives should adopt an approach of working closely with family members to make sure that women are cared for, and their autonomy respected while acknowledging the key role that family members play in achieving desirable care (Rosenberg et al., 2017). Some suggested phrases have been devised by Rosenberg et al. (2017) (Table 6.4) to assist healthcare professionals in exploring cultural perspectives, values and information needs of individuals using health services.

These strategies provide you with some ideas to start conversations with women and their families in a culturally sensitive way.

Practice Point

Ethical principles and moral values vary from culture to culture. Midwives use ethical principles in everyday clinical practise, which are guided by professional regulation. Every woman should be cared for ethically to ensure that she is treated fairly. Your care should consider her cultural beliefs and values when considering how to apply ethical principles.

Consequentialism

Consequentialism is an ethical theory that determines if something is right or wrong by what the consequences will be (Driver, 2011). One example of consequentialism is utilitarianism which judges consequences by a 'greatest good for the greatest number' standard (O'Gorman et al., 2013). Utilitarianism suggests that the best course of action is one in which happiness is maximised. The issue with consequentialism is at times; it may be difficult to determine the outcome in certain situations. If ethical action is when the outcome is considered to be a positive one by the majority of people, this is in conflict with treating the woman as an individual. For example, a midwife decides to spend most of her time performing postnatal checks on four women rather than use the time to spend on one woman who requires more time due to language difficulties. This results in the woman with the language barrier not receiving the same quality of care as other women, which may lead to missed problems. However, more good has been achieved for more women. On the other hand, the limited time provided to the woman with a language barrier may lead to an adverse outcome. You can justify practising in this way if no issues occur; however, once there is an issue, then consequentialism states this is an unethical practice. The NMC (2018) is not concerned with outcomes but rather with ensuring that midwives are doing the right thing.

TABLE 6.4 ■ **Phrases That Help Facilitate Exploration of Cultural Perspectives, Values and Information Needs**

Domain	Sample Phrases to Introduce the Conversation
Cultural perspectives and values	'Can you please tell me about your culture/community/faith?'
	'Can you tell me a little about yourself and what is important to you in your life?'
	'Can you tell me about your experiences in your home community in situations like this?'
	'When you think about what is ahead, what worries you most?'
Information delivery	'Different people/families like to hear information in different ways. Can you please share how you like to receive information?'
	'Are there particular people who you would like us to include when we share medical information?'
	'Are there particular people who you would like us not to include when we share medical information?'
Decision-making	'Can you please share with me how you and your family make decisions?'
	'When you have made medical decisions in the past, what were the circumstances that worked best for you?'
In cases of conflicting values (e.g., requests for collusion)	'When you think about telling [woman] about her [diagnosis], what worries you most?'
	'Would you mind telling me more about why you don't want [woman] to know about her [diagnosis]?'
	'When you think about what is ahead, what are you hoping for?'
	'Would it be okay if I told you what worries me about not telling her about her cancer?'

Adapted from Rosenberg, A.R., Starks, H., Unguru, Y., Feudtner, C., Diekema, D., 2017. Truth telling in the setting of cultural differences and incurable pediatric illness: a review. JAMA Pediatr. 171 (11), 1113–1119. https://doi.org/10.1001/jamapediatrics.2017.2568.

Problems arise when a midwife defends her actions based on consequentialism and not doing the right thing in the first instance.

Deontological Ethics

Deontological theories of ethics view the moral status of an action as dependent on its being in accord with a duty or rule of right action (Kranak, 2019). Hence, actions that obey these rules are ethical, while actions that do not are not ethical. Deontology comes from the Greek word *deon*, meaning 'duty'. This ethical theory is associated with the German philosopher, Immanuel Kant who was primarily concerned with doing the right thing simply because it was the right thing to do (Kranak, 2019). Kant divided his deontological beliefs between hypothetical and categorical imperatives (Misselbrook, 2013). Categorical imperatives are defined by Kant as moral and unconditional absolutes. In the context of healthcare, categorical imperatives would involve the health provider to consider if it would be acceptable for everyone to take the same action they were about to take (Cholbi, 2015); for example, a midwife acting in a way that any other midwife facing the same decision would consider the action to be justified and moral (Barrow and Khandhar, 2021).

You should acknowledge that each woman has her own predetermined goals and needs. If you consider your own personal agenda before that of the woman, then there is an ethical conflict. Maintaining this categorical imperative of practising in a way that would be acceptable by a majority of midwives respects the unique worth and dignity of the woman (Misselbrook, 2013; Mandal et al., 2016). Therefore, consideration of consequences is irrelevant in deontology and can be seen in the NMC (2018) Code, where there are rules which you should follow regardless of the possible outcomes.

Practice Point

An issue arises when an opinion on the right thing to do differs between you and the woman. Professional codes should influence your moral behaviour. The challenge is when there is conflict and dilemmas between your personal moral code, professional codes and the woman's morals, which may arise in clinical midwifery practice.

Ethical Dilemmas

In midwifery practice, ethical dilemmas may present due to the differences between the midwife's personal values and beliefs and the woman's. Ethical dilemmas are circumstances where decisions are made between two options that may be morally feasible but equally present a problem. These dilemmas may be increased when culture and religion are the reasons for these differences. Making decisions is an important skill for midwives, as well as advocating for women. When you are faced with a situation where there are no desirable actions or conflict between two actions, decision making and advocacy for the woman becomes difficult. You need to develop decision-making skills to deal with these ethical dilemmas. However, rule-based approaches to moral reasoning and ethical decision-making in the context of healthcare fails to recognise the importance of emotion in moral reasoning (Armstrong, 2007).

Moral uncertainty arises when an individual is unsure of what moral principle to adhere to or what values apply, or even what the moral problem is (Summers, 1985). Making a moral judgement involves the activity of thinking about whether something has a moral attribute (Cullity, 2011). This could be related to an action, an individual or even an organisation. Moral judgement that is constrained is said to be the basis for moral distress. You may face moral uncertainty if a judgement is made that an ethical principle should be applied which is against your morals. You may also face moral distress when you cannot find a solution to a problem or make a moral judgement but are unable to act on it.

Moral distress is different from other types of distress and has specific characteristics, the health professional having an awareness of their moral responsibility for ensuring patient wellbeing, a perception of powerlessness and anxieties associated with blame and a threat to the personal or professional integrity (Dudzinski, 2016). Moral distress can impact the care of women and may lead to the midwife's avoiding certain situations and interactions. In the face of moral distress, a midwife should be able to seek support regarding any dilemmas without the fear of being judged. Moral distress is more likely to arise within organisations where there are constraints on midwife's acting on their ethical principles, and there is no space for open and honest discussions. Moral distress can impact the ability to provide culturally competent care to women (Fig. 6.5).

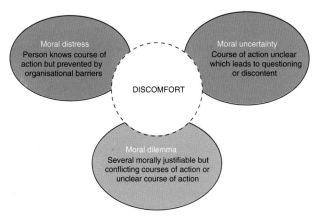

Fig. 6.5 Differences between moral distress, moral uncertainty and moral dilemma.

Practice Point

A key issue is when a midwife wishes to care for a woman ethically but has a moral dilemma or uncertainty about adopting the best stance. This is particularly relevant when you may not wish to prevent a woman from practising a cultural ritual, for example, but have a concern about the effect of the ritual on the woman's health. On the other hand, an issue may arise if you feel that the cultural ritual is harmless, but you are restrained from allowing the woman to practice her culture due to organisational policy.

Exercise

Review the following scenario to explore the issues that may arise when a cultural practice conflicts with evidence-based practice.

A midwife visits Lola and her baby in her home three days after spontaneous a vaginal delivery. The midwife notices that Lola is applying a herbal remedy to her baby's umbilical cord. On questioning, Lola explains to the midwife that this is standard cultural practice and is used to help the cord dry up more quickly.

Learning Activity

1. Is there an ethical dilemma in this scenario?
2. What could lead to moral uncertainty or distress?
3. How could the moral judgement of the midwife impact the cultural practice of Lola?

AUTONOMY OF WOMAN VERSUS AUTONOMY OF MIDWIFE

Culture determines the basis of potentiality for autonomy, as it sets boundaries for the level of autonomy for individuals within a society (Chirkov, 2017). Women from different cultures will therefore display autonomy differently. If it is accepted that humans are both cultural beings and are capable of autonomy and self-determination, then the question remains as to how cultural behaviour and a person's autonomy coexist and interact with each other (Park and Chirkov, 2020). Conflict in cultural beliefs and values may lead to the midwife's overriding the decisions made by women. As discussed earlier, a common ethical dilemma arises when respect for autonomy and cultural sensitivity collide; for instance, when a spouse makes an intervention decision for a woman, which the midwife may interpret as a bad decision. The midwife is faced with reconciling the sense that the woman had not freely exercised their autonomy with the desire to be culturally sensitive by respecting the value of community in a culture (Minkoff, 2014).

There have been concerns raised about the ethical principle of respect for autonomy and the apparent lack of adherence to this principle in practice in midwifery and maternity care services (Newnham and Kirkham, 2019). A suggestion that autonomy has become a hollowed-out practice referred to as rhetorical autonomy is debated. This term 'rhetorical autonomy' refers to the terms 'autonomy' and 'informed consent' regularly referred to in maternity care and underpins ethically sound maternity care practice. Yet, many women are denied both (Newnham and Kirkham, 2019). Women who do not question advice and treatment during pregnancy are believed to have been given autonomy. The reality is that if a woman is not given the opportunity or power to question practice that conflicts with her cultural beliefs and practices, then her autonomy is null and void. Newnham and Kirkham (2019) also propose that institutionalised birth as it is currently organised is inherently unethical; midwives and doctors are expected to place allegiance to hospital policy or cultural practices over respect for the wishes and needs of women.

The dignity and rights of the patients are given decent respect when patients are treated as independent individuals, regardless of their cultural and ethnic background (NMC, 2018). To fulfil the right of autonomy, clients should be informed with sufficient information regarding their health to support sound decision-making (Zhang and Min, 2020). However, lack of cultural awareness can lead to autonomy being taken away from the woman due to beliefs held by the midwife.

Autonomy may be shared by the family, and the individual in some cultures, and decisions may be made by elders or male family members. Paternalism stands on the opposite side of autonomy (Murgic et al., 2015). The point of paternalism in healthcare is that the health professional makes the decision in what is perceived to be the patient's best interests; this would include those who are capable of making the decision themselves (Sandman and Munthe, 2010). In midwifery practice, the woman is likely to heed the midwife's advice and ask what the best action regarding her pregnancy would be.

In contrast, to act maternalistically is for the midwife to decide for the woman based on a reasonable understanding of her preferences. The concept of maternalism allows for a more thorough assessment of the moral justification on acting in the woman's best interest (Sullivan, 2016). However, the danger here is assuming the woman's wishes are possibly based on incorrect information. Another danger is assuming that because a woman is from a particular background, she may wish for certain cultural practices. This fundamentally takes away a woman's right to make a decision regarding her pregnancy. You may want to ensure that a woman is given autonomy but need to consider if the choices she chooses are potentially harmful or a risk.

Maternity care stakeholders (e.g., clinicians, policymakers, insurers) can influence how pregnant women's rights during pregnancy and birth are upheld (Kruske et al., 2013). It is suggested that by focusing on patient autonomy to the detriment of beneficence, nonmaleficence and justice, there is a potential for services to become unjust as a whole and for individual decisions to regularly not be in the woman's interest (Lepping et al., 2016).

Practice Point

Autonomy is important in midwifery practice, and you should accept the impact of culture on women's decision-making. There needs to be cultural sensitivity regarding decisions that women make. You should respect her decisions, whether they are based on cultural beliefs or not. The midwife should take a stance to ensure that the woman is provided with the information needed to inform her decisions.

CONFLICT OF AUTONOMY AND BENEFICENCE

When there is a conflict between ethical principles, Gillon (2003) argues that autonomy should be considered above beneficence, nonmaleficence and justice. The principle of autonomy may often conflict with the principle of beneficence. Midwives who are attempting to show beneficence to women by using a paternalistic approach inadvertently breach autonomy. There may be cases whereby a midwife may limit information in a belief that this is what the woman wants to hear which takes away her right to make a decision based on all the necessary information. For example, if a midwife is aware that women from a particular culture would not accept genetic testing, this does not mean that information around screening for foetal abnormalities should be withheld. You should instead offer all the information in a culturally sensitive manner that acknowledges the woman's culture and her beliefs during any discussions. It is more important to respect the rights of the woman by promoting beneficence as well as autonomy.

CONFLICT OF BENEFICENCE AND JUSTICE

The principle of beneficence can also conflict with the principle of justice. Withholding information from a woman because there is concern from the midwife that she would not be able to understand such information is unethical. This may be due to language barriers or illiteracy. Illiteracy does not mean that a woman would not be able to understand health information. The decision from the midwife to tailor the information for the woman in an attempt to do good conflicts with justice, which is about fairness and equality. All women have equal rights in seeking healthcare and participating in their plan of care. Therefore, when all women are not afforded the same access to services and information regarding their pregnancy, this leads to a breach of justice. Unfortunately, there are incidents where women may not have interpreting services or written material available to them in a language they understand. The midwife is then faced with another dilemma of not being able to provide the woman with the required information.

CONFLICT OF BENEFICENCE AND NONMALEFICENCE

The principles of beneficence and nonmaleficence can often lead to conflict in midwifery practice. You should provide care to a woman in a culturally sensitive way; therefore, if adhering to beneficence, all available and evidence-based options should be offered. However, according to nonmaleficence, any care that provides harm should be ruled out.

To care for a woman ethically also requires cultural sensitivity, so consideration of cultural views is also needed. For example, if a woman was declining medication in pregnancy due to a cultural belief or value, then the midwife could adopt the ethical principle of nonmaleficence. This would be a culturally sensitive approach and leads to the woman feeling that she had control, support and respect for her culture. However, the ethical principle of beneficence would mean that you should explore all treatment options with the woman and work towards a consensus. This could lead to the woman feeling that her wishes and decision are challenged, leading to stress and lack of satisfaction with the maternity service. Such factors will impact the midwife/woman relationship.

These dilemmas of doing good but preventing harm can arise in many situations where the woman wants to follow a cultural practice, but there is a conflict with recommended midwifery care practice.

Screening for genetic disorders is a routine practice during pregnancy. All women should be offered screening regardless of their culture or religion. Please read the following scenario.

Exercise

Ari is attending for a booking interview at 11 weeks gestation. The midwife has discussed the screening for foetal abnormalities with Ari and has asked for permission to take blood for this. Ari has declined any screening and does not wish to know if her baby may have a higher chance of a foetal abnormality. She explains that in her culture, whether her baby is affected or not, she would continue the pregnancy. However, Ari does wish to have the early pregnancy scan, including a nuchal translucency test. The midwife knows that the pregnancy scan is also part of the screening for foetal abnormalities.

Learning Activity

1. What ethical principles can be applied to this scenario and why?
2. What steps should the midwife take to ensure that the ethical principles are applied?

Other Moral or Behavioural Concerns

CONSENT AND CAPACITY

The woman has a right to choose to adhere to a cultural practice or belief, which is safeguarded by the principle of autonomy (Taylor, 2013). The midwife faced with a dilemma of whether a cultural practice should be facilitated needs to be cognisant of the law. The Mental Capacity Act (MCA) (2005) safeguards the right for a woman to decline treatment or intervention. In some cases, lack of cultural awareness or sensitivity and lack of knowledge may lead to a midwife's believing that the woman does not have mental capacity solely because she continues to refuse an intervention even if it may harm her baby. It is accepted by law that women have the capacity to make decisions about their pregnancy, and if deemed otherwise, it must be supported by the evidence (MCA, 2005).

Informed consent is not merely pushing information at a woman. It is an opportunity to initiate a dialogue between health professionals and their clients in which both attempt to arrive at a mutually satisfactory course of action. Informed consent should result in making a shared decision (Allesee and Gallagher, 2011).

A decision made with full capacity must be respected even if it appears unwise or irrational. Where capacity is questioned, Section 2 of the MCA (2005) guides professionals. The legislation is quite clear in stating that lack of capacity cannot be established by reference to: '(a) a person's age or appearance, or (b) a condition of his, or an aspect of his behaviour, which might lead others to make unjustified assumptions about his capacity' (MCA, 2005).

Capacity is a shared phenomenon in some cultures that cannot be strictly enjoyed or expressed by the individual except when the person is 'alienated' from the family (Norman, 2015). For example, in African cultures, there is the social expectation that elders and educated professionals such as a doctor probably know best, compared to the average person in health matters (Norman, 2015).

You should always judge that a woman is competent, and she should always be provided with an opportunity to give her consent before any care is provided. This consent should always be voluntary and free from any coercion. For the consent to be 'informed', it is important that the woman understands what you have said.

Effectively, consent can render physical contact lawful, whereby a woman's consent makes touching legally permitted (Mason and Laurie, 2013). In cultures where the family functions as a single unit and 'family autonomy' is higher than the person's autonomy, issues can arise around informed consent. Family units in some groups of society would want to play a pivotal role in decision-making when risks of treatment involving their family member are explained (Norman, 2015).

Complications may arise when a woman lives in a culture where deference to authority figures or elders and non-individual decision-making is the cultural norm (Di Mattia, 2008). In this situation, you should be aware of the importance of this joint decision-making to the woman. A worry you may have is that consent is coerced by family pressure. However, you should understand and accept the concept of informed consent and autonomy in different cultures.

Review the following scenario, which provides further explanation of this.

Exercise

Suna is in labour and has made no progress, resulting in the midwife asking for a review by an obstetrician. The obstetrician advises Suna that intervention is needed as she has made no progress for several hours. Despite this information, Suna does not wish to have any intervention and declines consent for a caesarean section. Suna has her mother and partner in the room who tell the obstetrician and midwife that vaginal birth is preferred.

Learning Activity

1. What are the ethical principles that should be considered in this scenario?
2. What other information should the midwife seek from Suna and her family about the choice made?

Now review the following scenario to see how cultural sensitivity and ethical sensitivity has been used.

The midwife asks Suna whether there are any cultural reasons why vaginal birth is preferred. Suna and her family explain that giving birth naturally is more culturally acceptable as a caesarean birth is believed to lower the status of motherhood. Despite further extended discussion from the obstetrician and midwife of the potential impact of no intervention on the baby, Suna still declines. The midwife asks if there is anyone she can contact who can help Suna and her family make a decision. An elder from Suna's community is contacted who attends and hears the reasons from the obstetrician and midwife why intervention is needed. The obstetrician and the midwife provide privacy for Suna and the elder to make a decision. Soon after, Suna gives her consent for a caesarean section.

Practice Point

Understanding how women make decisions in different cultures requires insight into the importance of family and community. Ethical dilemmas can arise when midwives face scenarios where it may seem that the decision to consent for a treatment is a joint decision. However, applying ethical principles ensures that the woman's cultural wishes are respected and heard.

DECISION-MAKING

The quality of the care provided by midwives is directly related to the quality of the decision-making process (Jefford, 2012). Midwives have to make decisions every day and these are affected by moral and ethical principles. Poor decision-making is a theme evident in confidential enquiries and audit reports, indicating that poor clinical decision-making contributes to poor maternal and neonatal outcomes (Draper et al., 2015; Knight et al., 2015). Therefore, the importance of good decision-making should not be underestimated. Cheyne et al. (2012) discuss three elements in the decision-making process of midwives: the *assessment* (the professional's judgement of the level of risk), the *decision* (the choice between possible courses of action) and the *decision threshold* (the professional's threshold when linking the judgement and the decision). Hence, a certain level of skill and knowledge is required to undertake effective decision-making. More importantly, decisions made by the midwife need to always consider the risk or potential harm to the woman. It is suggested that the primary source of variation is in the personal *decision thresholds* of professionals (Cheyne et al., 2012).

Daemers et al. (2017) identify five themes that influence a midwife's everyday clinical decision-making: the pregnant woman as a whole person, the midwife as a whole person, sources of knowledge, collaboration between maternity care professionals and organisation of care. Several factors impact the 'midwife as a whole' making decisions about women in her care, including women centredness and shared decision-making. The focus on the woman is vital in this aspect as considering her cultural values and beliefs should be critical in shared decision-making (Fig. 6.6).

Shared decision-making is supported in the guidance produced by National Institute for Health and Care Excellence (NICE, 2017), which states that the following elements should be present:
- Care or treatment options are fully explored, along with their risks and benefits
- Different choices available to the patient are discussed
- A decision is reached together with a health and social care professional.

This signifies that you should make an effort to ensure that a decision is reached together with the woman; however, it can only be achieved once she has all the information. In women who have limited English or a language barrier, it is accepted that appropriate translation services should be acquired and appropriate written information provided. Ethically, unless all communication and language barriers are addressed, shared decision-making has not been achieved.

Shared decision-making has several advantages, including empowering the woman to make informed choices, the ability for the midwife to tailor care to meet the needs of the woman, and understanding what is important to the woman. To engage in shared decision-making honestly requires that a midwife acknowledges (1) their responsibility to the woman (respect for patient autonomy), (2) their responsibility to be true to their own clinical judgement about the best interests of the woman (beneficence), (3) their accountability to society (distributive justice) and (4) the uncertainty of the evidence (Christine and Kaldjian, 2013).

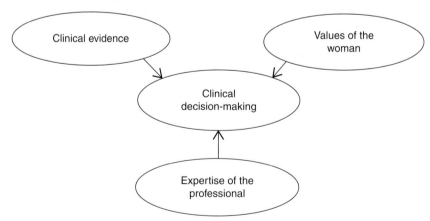

Fig. 6.6 Factors influencing the clinical decision-making of midwives. (Reproduced with permission from Daemers et al., 2017. Factors influencing the clinical decision-making of midwives: a qualitative study. BMC Pregnancy Childbirth. 17 (1), 345.)

Shared decision-making promotes the ethical principle of respect for patient autonomy by empowering the woman (Elwyn et al., 2012). Regarding communicating evidence, beneficence also supports efforts to promote a patient's understanding of the treatment options offered as there is a relation between autonomy and beneficence since one of the ways to act for a patient's good is to enhance their autonomy (Christine and Kaldjian, 2013).

In collective societies found in Africa, Asia and the Middle East, family-facilitated and collective decision-making processes are consistent with the belief that an individual is an amalgamation of herself with family and society. A good practice is to make sure all decision-making is underpinned by ethical consideration (Jones, 2005). This ensures that decisions that are made safeguard women against physical and emotional harm. The midwife should encourage choice and involvement as this supports the ethical principle of autonomy (Cooke, 2005). The aim should be to practice cultural safety by balancing the power between the woman and the midwife, which, as already discussed, protects her cultural identity. Access to information must be emphasised both during the process of decision-making and after that. In cultures where the family rather than the individual makes decisions, this practice must be respected if this is the woman's request. Patients and their families should share decisions with practitioners and receive additional information (Laidsaar-Powell et al., 2016).

Read the following exercise to further highlight the importance of shared decision-making.

Exercise

A woman is in labour and is accompanied by her mother and husband. She is requesting pain relief. The midwife discusses pain relief options with the woman, who asks her mother and husband what their views are. The mother of the woman and the husband do not wish for an epidural to be given. The midwife considers everyone's views and a decision is reached that everyone is happy with.

Learning Activity

1. What do you think could be the possible ethical issues the midwife may have with sharing information with the woman's family?
2. What cultural factors could have influenced the woman's behaviour?
3. What could have been the outcome if shared decision-making had not been facilitated?

DECISIONAL CONFLICT

Stacey et al. (2008) discuss the concept of "decisional conflict" as the gap between what midwives believe women should know and what women want to know. Suggesting that midwives, in some incidences, will take on a paternalistic role when making decisions that may deem to be unethical practice as the basis of informed consent should be to provide all the necessary information to the woman. The exclusion of information by health professionals has been confirmed by other studies and introduced as the major obstacle in decision-making (Camerini and Schulz, 2016). However, it is argued that if the midwife provides information, regardless of the woman's identity and values, this is likely to confuse her and does not facilitate decision-making (Stacey et al., 2008). There are also issues with treating all women the same. Stacey et al. (2008) state that the assumption of "one size fits all contexts" neglects personal differences. It is believed that a woman who makes a decision that is based on their personal values and beliefs will readily accept the consequences of their choices. The skill required here is to understand the woman's viewpoint, be aware and sensitive of her culture and be prepared to explain all the woman's questions.

MODELS OF DECISION-MAKING

Barber (2012) looked at several decision-making models and identified two key approaches: the analytical/rational approach and the intuitive/experimental approach. It is argued that midwifery reasoning is a combination of the two approaches. The analytical/rational approach to decision-making fits within a knowledge framework and is logical and systematic. It is focused on the analysis of all facts and the development and testing of hypotheses. However, the intuitive/ experimental approach to decision-making relies more on the midwife's intuition and previous experience. Intuition is the process by which knowledge, skills and self-awareness are combined to make more than the sum of their parts (Barnfather, 2013). Intuition in midwifery practice has been explored by (Olsson and Adolfsson, 2012) and linked to a broadening and deepening knowledge, skills and experience. As expertise increases, so does the role of intuitive decision-making. The use of intuition may be risky, as it can be used in the face of incomplete information. Concerning cultural safety, intuition should not be used to determine the right decision for a woman; the midwife should acquire all the facts from the woman. Intuition can cause a midwife to engage in intuitive judgement prematurely, however, clinical judgement should be both ethical and evidenced-based (Muoni, 2012).

Please review the exercise on which provides an example of intuitive decision-making.

Exercise

Clare is conducting an antenatal assessment for a woman who is 24 weeks pregnant and having her first baby. The woman has discussed with Clare what will happen during the birth and wants further information on this. On checking the woman's notes, there has been no discussion of parent education classes being offered. Clare asks the woman if classes were offered to which she replies 'No'.

Learning Activity

1. What may have influenced the decision made by the midwife who did the booking interview not to offer antenatal classes?
2. How could intuition have influenced the midwife's decision not to offer antenatal classes?
3. What should Clare do now to address the wishes conveyed by the woman?

Practice Point

The previous scenario highlights the importance of not using intuition to decide what care or services to provide to women. Often midwives will use prior experience with intuition to assign care to a woman and does not consider her personal preferences. In the next section, informed consent will be discussed, emphasising the importance of providing the woman with the appropriate information to facilitate her decision-making.

INFORMED CONSENT

Informed consent is an ethical requirement. Obtaining informed consent involves informing the woman about her rights, the purpose of any care provided and the potential risks and benefits. Informed consent is said to support individual autonomy. The importance of informed consent is that it prevents the chance of a woman being coerced or deceived into accepting treatment or any care. On the other hand, lack of information may prevent the woman from asking for a service or care that she prefers. The origins of informed consent in healthcare can be traced back to the ethics of research involving human subjects in response to experiments conducted during World

War 1. In 1946, the Nuremberg Code was developed, which stated that the voluntary consent of human subjects is essential and that experiments should be conducted in a manner to avoid all unnecessary physical and mental suffering and injury (Showalter, 2012).

Respect for an autonomous individual requires acknowledging her 'right to make choices, hold views and take actions based on her personal values and beliefs' (Beauchamp and Childress, 2013). Information should be culturally adjusted, taking local factors into account. These might include degrees of illiteracy, native dialects of ethnic minorities, a lack of suitable vocabulary, a preference for communal decision-making and stigmatisation by local authorities if people do not sign (Guerrier et al., 2012). The midwife's role in ensuring that women are giving informed consent should consider her cultural wishes and desires. If there is conflict between the woman's preferences and what usually is available, you should take steps to accommodate the woman's needs.

Practice Point

Often in clinical practice, there may be a conflict between what the organisation has to offer and what the woman desires. This could be very simple such as appointment times that conflict with cultural or religious festivals or wishing to have a female attendant. You can compromise in these circumstances and adjust plans of care. Advocating for a woman is important to ensure her wishes are heard and respected. When this does not occur then, it is reasonable to suggest you have not supported the woman.

INFORMED CHOICE

Informed choice is defined as a right to make an uncoerced and informed decision (Beauchamp and Childress, 2013). 'Choice' is not like 'consent' as it is not linked with another person's suggestion. Healthcare professionals approach the issue of informed choice, asking by individuals to choose from a 'menu of choices' rather than give consent to a particular suggestion (Spaeth, 2010). For example, if you are offering a woman the choice of hospital or home birth, she will consider your remarks and make a choice. The woman may choose to have a home birth, but she has not consented to have a home birth. You should present all the choices available as well as provide detail and perhaps recommend a particular choice. When the woman *chooses*, the midwife is perceived as an advisor who is more knowledgeable than the woman (Spaeth, 2010).

Informed choice is considered an ethical principle that guides 'woman-centred care'. There has been a large amount of literature on how to facilitate informed choice. Unfortunately, the pursuit of promoting women's autonomy and providing a woman with the care that aligns with their culture and personal values leads to complexity. Women are being offered less choice depending on the clinical situation and the midwife and researchers have argued that informed choice, in particular, is an illusion (Jenkinson et al., 2016).

The literature suggests that to make an informed choice, individuals need to deliberate about relevant information by evaluating the 'advantages and disadvantages of all the possible courses of action, in accordance with their beliefs' (Bekker, 2006). Woman's views of how they view their body plays a very important part in the choices they make. The socio-cultural and religious context is different for every woman. This impacts the choices that women make, which may seem unreasonable to the midwife. As discussed in previous chapters, the importance of cultural safety ensures that power imbalances do not occur. If the midwife's cultural beliefs and values differ from the woman's, this may lead to the midwife inadvertently only offering the choices s/he wishes the woman to make. Women may, therefore, have fewer opportunities to engage in the dynamic processes required for shared decision-making (Nieuwenhuijze et al., 2014). Informed choice should be the product of shared decision-making. Hence, in the absence of shared decision-making informed choice is not facilitated leading to a woman not being given the human rights she is entitled to.

Midwives need to accept that a woman may listen to all the advice she is offered, but the choice she makes may not necessarily be the one that a midwife is comfortable with. In other cases, a midwife may think that the woman is not of sound mind because the choice she has made conflicts with policy or professional views. For example, declining screening for Down's syndrome or diagnostic testing in the event of abnormal results. Nolan (2011) states that it is unreasonable and offensive to consider any choice as inappropriate or stupid if it is informed.

Informed choice is recognised and accepted as an important aspect of ethical healthcare (Ballantyne et al., 2006). However, when there are choices made by a woman that pose some extent of risk, ethically, the midwife may feel obliged to counteract that risk. The report Better Births (NHS England, 2020) identified that the importance of choice and the safety of both mother and baby being paramount could cause conflict. Thompson (2013), in a small qualitative study, described that the increasing social and cultural values of convenience and control in Western society correlates with questions about women's ability to birth and professional's clinical skills. Thompson (2013) also identified that midwives experienced discomfort when women chose care outside of the guidelines, and midwives raised concerns about the reality of informed choice in some specific groups. For example, facilitating informed choice with non-English speaking women around treatment for a condition was particularly a challenge, even when using interpreters and translated information leaflets. This occurs in the event that there are no words for the tested-for conditions in their first language (Ahmed et al., 2013).

Midwives should also recognise that facilitating informed choice involves ensuring that the woman 'has sufficient time to make an informed decision' (NICE, 2021). Time limitations impact the midwife delivering all the information that the woman requires. This is again particularly relevant to women who have language barriers or health illiteracy. Even with the presence of a professional interpreter, time limitations impact the quality of the information delivered to the woman. There is also a potential for midwives to influence women's choices. Midwives have admitted that they have focused on enabling women to make informed choices based on their own understandings of the information, available options and their own values (Ahmed et al., 2013). However, autonomous informed choices can be enhanced by organisation factors such as allowing increased time during clinical interactions and educating health professionals on how to accommodate women with language barriers (Ahmed et al., 2013).

ACCOUNTABILITY

Accountability means being responsible for your actions regardless of the actions of others. It is evident within the NMC (2018) Code that the midwife has a professional and legal obligation to be accountable. The purpose of holding midwives to account for their actions is to ensure the safety of the public, expectant mothers and their babies and to provide redress to those who have been harmed (Griffith, 2011). Accountability can lead to a midwife being transparent about her practice, using evidence-based, informed decisions and engaging with women to offer informed choices. The midwife's experience and any external factors such as the culture of the unit and support from managers impact accountability (Fowler, 2008). However, you have an individual responsibility to act in such a way as to protect the women in your care regardless of external factors. Accountability has several functions, according to Griffith (2011), that ensures a midwife continues to practice with responsibility and accountability, which protects the woman (Table 6.5).

You are accountable for providing each woman with a high standard of care. This includes the need to protect her cultural identity and facilitate her cultural needs. You are also accountable for seeking out information on the woman's culture, discussing with the woman her cultural preferences, ensuring that any care provided does not seriously conflict with the woman's culture and offering culturally sensitive alternatives. Midwives, as well as being accountable for any care

TABLE 6.5 ■ **Three Functions of Accountability**

A protective function	Protects women from any acts or omissions of the midwife that might cause harm. Midwives whose practice has fallen below the required standard can have their conduct and competence questioned
A deterrent function	Authorities can hold midwives accountable by using sanctions to discourage them from acting in a way that would be considered misconduct or unlawful
A regulatory function	The NMC regulatory framework makes it clear what standard of conduct and competence is required by a registered midwife
An educative function	Midwives can be called to account and asked to justify their actions and be subject to having their cases heard in public with a view to reassuring women that only the highest standards of practice will be tolerated. This public examination of a midwife's conduct acts as a learning tool for other midwives to learn from the mistakes and misconduct of others

Reproduced with permission from Griffith, R., 2011. Understanding accountability in midwifery practice: Key concepts. Br. J. Midwifery. 19 (5), 327–328.

provided to the woman, should also be aware of their limitations and the need to escalate any issues or concerns. Accountability should include addressing any disparities in healthcare, systematic racism, stereotyping and any actions that oppress and marginalise women.

ADVOCACY

The term 'advocacy' stems etymologically from the Latin word '*advocatus*', which is the past participle of '*ad vocare*' which means to (ad) call (vocare) as a witness or representative (Watson and Connor, 2017). The role of advocacy in midwifery practice is needed to ensure women are treated fairly. The NMC Code states it is the responsibility of midwives to 'act as an advocate for the vulnerable, challenging poor practice and discriminatory attitudes and behaviour relating to their care' (NMC, 2018).

Evidence has revealed that advocacy can range from supporting the woman in decision-making to more assertive actions such as 'standing up' for or whistleblowing on behalf of the woman (Hanks, 2008). Curtin (1979) and Fowler (1989) proposed a holistic view of advocacy expressed in five categories: moral–ethical, legal, political, spiritual and substitutive (Table 6.6).

It has been advised by Association for Improvements in the Maternity Services (AIMS, 2012) a need for midwives who can differentiate between being coercive agents, enforcers of the system and being advocates for the women within it. The challenge of respecting a woman's cultural wishes and adhering to unit policy is an ongoing issue. You should focus on supporting women who make decisions about birth that practitioners do not necessarily agree with, as decisions

TABLE 6.6 ■ **Examples of Categories of Advocacy**

Legal advocate	The midwife guards the woman's rights to competent care, to reject care, informed consent and privacy
Moral–ethical advocate	The midwife upholds the woman's values in decision-making
Political advocate	The midwife facilitates equal access to healthcare
Spiritual advocate	The midwife provides access to spiritual support and reassurance
Substitutive advocate	The midwife protects the interests of women who are incapable of speaking for themselves

about birth are not child protection issues (AIMS, 2012). The expectation is that professionals understand the nature of advocacy to recognise the risk of a power imbalance between the patient and the caregiver and provide dignified, respectful care (Martin, 2015). However, it is argued that despite being well-intentioned, a hasty and uneducated willingness to accept something as a cultural good can still cause significant harm (Muaygil, 2018). The ability of a midwife to advocate depends on several personal or organisational factors. It is indicated that a midwife's age, educational level and work setting could influence advocacy (Kubsch et al., 2004). A midwife without cultural awareness or knowledge may stereotype unconsciously, causing inappropriate advocacy. Therefore, advocacy is a skill that needs to be developed and revisited by ongoing training for midwives.

In the next section, scenarios are provided on the different categories of advocacy.

Legal Advocacy

Lola has decided to continue a pregnancy with a baby who has confirmed Edwards syndrome, a condition that has a poor prognosis. Usually, most women would opt for a termination of pregnancy, but Lola, after receiving advice, does not wish to do so, as it is her personal and cultural wish. Members of the team question Lola as to why she is continuing a pregnancy that is likely to result in intrauterine or neonatal death. A midwife is allocated to caseload Lola and ensures she has her serial scans and appointments as required for a high-risk pregnancies. The midwife as a legal advocate safeguards Lola's right to refuse a termination and ensures she receives the appropriate amount of pregnancy surveillance. Lola was therefore empowered by the midwife, who reduced the organisational control caused by policy and professional views.

Moral-Ethical Advocacy

Jana has expressed to her midwife that she does not want to be induced at 42 weeks and has voiced this to her consultant, who has arranged admission in any case. The midwife communicates this to the obstetrician on call and helps Jana explain that labour induction conflicts with her cultural values. The midwife acts as a cultural broker between the woman and the healthcare system. In this way, Jana's right to autonomous decision-making and self-determination is protected.

Political Advocacy

Midwives often lack the power to change maternity services that do not facilitate advocacy for women and their families. A union representative spoke at a maternity unit meeting, stating that staffing ratios were impacting midwives' ability to work safely in the workplace, which in turn impacted the woman's safety. Due to this changes were made to increase staffing ratios and ensure that there was an appropriate skill mix. This stance enhanced the safety of the women utilising the maternity service.

Spiritual Advocacy

Merna has just delivered her baby, and her husband wishes to say a special prayer for the baby before she breastfeeds. Even though the midwife needs to do checks on the baby, she allows this to happen. The midwife has respected Merna's right to undertake a spiritual rite and protect her culture. This demonstrates a holistic approach to midwifery care that does not just focus on physical tasks. The midwife has facilitated Merna in practicing her culture.

Substitutive Advocacy

Huda has an elective caesarean section, and the midwife is preparing her for the surgery. Huda does not speak English and usually wears the hijab according to her Muslim faith. Being aware of this, the midwife takes care that Huda is allowed to cover her head in theatre and ensures that she is not unnecessarily exposed by communicating Huda's wishes to the theatre team during the whole of the surgery. In this way, the midwife has respected Huda by maintaining dignity and privacy.

Women require midwives to be on their side when they feel vulnerable amid a largely impersonal system (AIMS, 2012). You should support the woman and not expect her to conform to the organisational rules and policies if it conflicts with her personal beliefs and values. Often midwives find it difficult to speak up for the woman, and this may be due to a lack of cultural knowledge of the importance of some cultural practices and rituals. Midwives should be able to have sensitive discussions with a woman on their cultural wishes and needs so that they understand the woman's views. In addition, midwives need to be able to advocate for the woman if there is a conflict between pregnancy care and a cultural practice or belief. It is particularly important for you to advocate for women who may not be able to self-advocate due to language barriers, lack of knowledge and low health literacy. However, it is difficult to advocate for the woman if there is a lack of awareness of cultural factors that may impact the woman's wishes.

Practice Point

As advocates, you need to both understand the culture of your client whilst also understanding the context and limitations of the maternity services and act as a bridge between the two.

The following section discusses the organisational factors that can impact midwives practising ethically.

Organisational Impact on Ethical Practice

ORGANISATIONAL CULTURE

Organisational culture is considered a key determinant in the quality of care provided (Davies et al., 2007). There are various definitions for organisational culture ranging from shared beliefs and values, which provide individuals with rules for behaviour, to the importance of an individual's cultural experiences to the cultural community (Mannion and Davies, 2018). Organisational culture in maternity units impacts maternal and neonatal health and good midwifery practice. Hence, if the organisational culture is flawed, consequently care provision is also flawed.

There are several reports of healthcare institutions where organisational culture has led to poor care outcomes. Three of the most widely known examples occurred in the Mid Staffordshire (Francis, 2010), Morecambe Bay Foundation Trusts (Kirkup, 2015) and the Shrewsbury and Telford Hospital NHS Trust (Ockenden, 2020) in the UK. The public inquiry reports evidenced communication failures between the workforce, institutions and regulatory bodies that contributed to patient morbidity and mortality and the continuation of an inadequate operating workplace. This included severe workforce shortages, a lack of compassionate and quality care and a failure to take patient, relative and staff complaints seriously.

The report by Francis (2010), in its investigation of cases of substandard care, recommended a 'fundamental culture change' to improve the safety of services – making a clear link between organisational culture and the organisation's performance. The Morecambe Bay Investigation (Kirkup, 2015) provided a severe picture of poor working relationships between different professional groups, unwillingness to question poor practices and zealous pursuit of professional ideology resulting in a dysfunctional organisational culture. Inadequate levels of care within the maternity services and opportunities to learn from incidents and improve services were identified in the Ockenden report (Ockenden, 2020).

In a scoping review by Frith et al. (2014) of organisational culture in maternity units, it was found that a common theme running through the research findings was significant organisational barriers to practising 'proper' midwifery care. Midwives felt that they were part of a subculture who were unable to practise according to their philosophy of care (Frith et al., 2014). This can lead to poor ethical practices that influence how women are cared for. Ethical principles in healthcare organisations lay a foundation for quality care. The most pressing organisational ethics issues are resource allocation, clinical issues, staff morale distress linked to the organisation's moral climate and conflicts of interest (Silva et al., 2008). When priority is not given to these issues, it is fair to say that ethical standards decline.

Unethical workplace behaviours can have far-reaching consequences – job losses, risks to life and health and psychological damage to individuals and groups (Lindebaum et al., 2017). In addition, emotions, including moral emotions, may be suppressed in an organisation, which negatively impacts women's care (Lindebaum, 2012).

Practice Point

As discussed in previous sections, you should be mindful of how organisational culture influences care provision and impacts women. Steps can be taken to change poor organisational cultures, but to what degree this can be done individually is questioned. The following sections look at particular aspects of organisational culture that impact ethical care.

WORKPLACE INFLUENCE ON MIDWIVES GIVING WOMEN AUTONOMY

The workplace can impact a midwife's autonomous practice due to persisting domination of the medical model (Sonmezer, 2021). Since the creation of the midwifery profession, power relationships between midwives and obstetricians have created professional conflict, leaving midwives feeling oppressed and obstetricians feeling like their medical authority is disregarded (Reiger, 2008). The ability for midwives to provide support to women to make decisions about their care is further hindered by the culture and environment that midwives work in (Jefford et al., 2016).

Newnham and Kirkham (2019) identified that midwives' and doctors' compliance with guidelines and institutionalised practice is considered more important than women's choice and is unethical. leading to the choices of women being controlled by health professionals (Fig. 6.7). In addition, the fear that litigation creates for staff working within maternity services results in changes in practice, including defensiveness and increased reliance on medical permission (Robertson and Thomson, 2016). Health professionals often feel pressured to encourage women to comply with hospital policies and routines or are pressured to withhold information or present information in ways that do not challenge women's prior thinking (Lothian, 2009). Unfortunately, the focus on guideline compliance neglects care provision that is in the best interests of the woman (Robertson and Thomson, 2016), contradicting the professional duty to prioritise people by recognising diversity and individual choice (NMC, 2018).

Clinical governance frameworks should support the role of the midwife as an advocate. The components of clinical governance described by Braithwaite and Travaglia (2008) includes the promotion of safety and quality and the development of clinical governance structures to improve safety and quality. An ineffective clinical governance framework with no clear communication channels disables patient advocacy and creates a workplace culture that prevents openness.

BLAME CULTURE

When things go wrong, it is important that there is open and transparent communication so that adverse outcomes can be managed and, more importantly, prevented. Good ethical practice can be affected within organisations that have a blame culture. If midwives are free from the fear of blame, there is the likelihood that they may be more likely to be open about errors; this enables organisations to identify issues and rectify any problems (Provera et al., 2010).

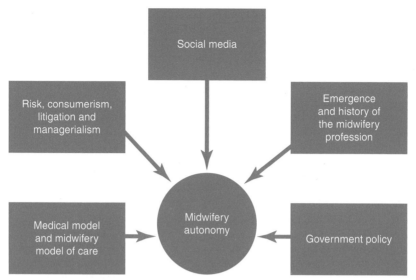

Fig. 6.7 Influences on midwife autonomy. (Reproduced with permission from Sonmezer, E., 2021. Professional autonomy for midwives in the contemporary UK maternity system: Part 2. Br. J. Midwifery. 29 (1), 19–25.)

A no-blame culture has several benefits such as increasing patient safety and improving standards of care and is achieved by error-reporting procedures that are 'safe' for individuals, with staff actively encouraged to record and report any problems and 'near-misses' (Gronewold et al., 2013). In addition, processes should be in place for staff to reflect on inclusive errors and systems for identifying and implementing improvements are communicated positively and openly (Lupton and Warren, 2018). These elements rely on employees having certain values and moral qualities and a willingness to be open about mistakes, which should not be abused by managers, and a culture of involvement and sharing knowledge across hierarchies (Lupton and Warren, 2018).

Apart from the impact of a blame culture on ethical practice, if managers and employees have to work in an environment where they are blamed for failure, innovation and risk-taking are likely to be stifled (Schilling and Kluge, 2009). Hence, midwives are kept on a tight lead regarding facilitating women's choices or advocating for women's autonomy. A blame culture inadvertently suppresses the cultural safety of women.

BARRIERS TO WHISTLEBLOWING

The benefits of internal whistleblowing or speaking up is significant in healthcare (Rauwolf and Jones, 2019). There is no question that the exposure of poor practice can lead to improvements in the quality of care. Midwives have a responsibility to raise concerns about the safety of women and babies and unethical or illegal conduct. Whistleblowing is an act of advocacy that can be justified from many ethical perspectives (Grant, 2002; Kline, 2006). This includes the ethical principles of nonmalificence and truth-telling. Midwives who fail to whistleblow about poor ethical behaviour or practices may be seen to be practising unethically. Lachman (2008) further states that failure to act and report concerns breaches professional codes and violates basic virtues, hence why midwives should adopt whistleblowing as an advocacy role.

The UK whistleblowing legislation is situated within the Employment Rights Act 1996; the legislation sets out the requirements for any disclosures to be protected under the law but does not guarantee protection (Watson and Connor, 2017). Therefore, due to this lack of protection, midwives may fear to whistleblow due to the potential impact of being mistreated by their managers and employing organisations. Whistleblowers have experienced bullying and intimidation, job losses, loss of relationships; the threat of legal action; and all the financial, emotional and social losses that follow (Patrick, 2012).

A comprehensive and independent overview of the situation within the NHS has recognised the challenges and consequences for actual or potential whistleblowers (Francis, 2010). Organisations that do not facilitate whistleblowing can create serious consequences for service users and staff well-being (Rauwolf and Jones, 2019). For example, racism and discrimination in the NHS show that there are issues with health professionals not practising ethically and that this is behaviour is not being challenged.

SYSTEMIC RACISM

Systemic racism can be defined as the collective failure of an organisation to provide appropriate and professional services to individuals because of their culture or ethnic origin (Lim et al., 2021). Racism in healthcare is an ethical issue that impacts racial, religious and ethnic groups (Danis et al., 2016). When reviewing the main ethical principles, there is a serious conflict between what constitutes good ethical practice and racism. Unfair treatment of human beings based on race and ethnicity demonstrates that racism is primarily a subject of ethics (Elias and Paradies, 2021). Explicit forms of systemic racism that emerged with the rise of European colonisation, industrial capitalism and the Atlantic slave trade continue to manifest in 21st-century Western societies (Elias and Paradies, 2021). Acknowledgement of this fact is needed by healthcare services as treatment of individuals who are deemed to be different or in a minority population has continued from these historical events. This is supported by research that has reported evidence of implicit and explicit racist beliefs, emotions, or practices among healthcare providers (Maina et al., 2018).

One ethical flaw of racism is disrespect to individuals based on their ethnicity or race (Glasgow, 2009). Disrespect in maternity services is highlighted as being a transgression of a woman's human rights. Services that are geared towards a majority population or does not provide for a woman to maintain her cultural identity is a breach of autonomy. Nonmaleficence and beneficence conflict with racist behaviour as not causing harm or doing good is arguably not a trait in racist behaviour. Racism also leads to unfairness and is ethically indefensible as it fundamentally stamps on justice, equality and human dignity by imposing bias and inequity based on unfair socially constructed human differences (Elias and Paradies, 2021).

Organisations that deny the existence of systemic racism legitimises and justifies poor ethical behaviour. Unfortunately, failing to acknowledge the presence of systemic racism is a failure to address why this occurs. Turning a blind eye to systemic racism allows unfair treatment of individuals to continue and flourish in some cases. Racism can manifest in several forms in maternity services, including lack of choice, poor advocacy, poor communication, inappropriate interpretation services, lack of privacy and confidentiality and failure to listen to concerns of women. Barriers to healthcare that lead to inequitable access and disregard of the cultural needs of minority groups create disparities and systemic racism (Better, 2008).

Practice Point

The organisational ethical issues have been highlighted as being vital to you practising ethically. Even more relevant is the role that you play in ensuring that your midwifery practice is ethical. A midwife who can meet these challenges embraces the autonomous nature of a midwife and the importance of being with women.

1. Think about how you practise ethically in your clinical area.
2. Is there a particular ethical principle that raises issues in your clinical practice?
3. How important is utilising ethical principles in midwifery practice to care outcomes for women.
4. Are there any ethical principles that you feel should be considered first before any other?

References

Ahmed, S., Bryant, L.D., Cole, P., 2013. Midwives' perceptions of their role as facilitators of informed choice in antenatal screening. Midwifery 29 (7), 745–750.

Aksoy, S., Tenik, A., 2002. The 'four principles of bioethics' as found in 13th century Muslim scholar Mawlana's teachings. BMC Med. Ethics 3 (1), 1–7.

Allesee, L., Gallagher, C.M., 2011. Pregnancy and protection: the ethics of limiting a pregnant woman's participation in clinical trials. J. Clin. Res. Bioeth. 2 (108), 1000108. https://doi.org/10.4172/2155-9627.1000108.

Alperovitch, A., Dreifuss-Netter, F.D.R., Dickele, A.M., Gaudray, P., Coz, P.L., Rouvillois, P., Roux, M., Waquet, P., 2009. Ethical issues raised by a possible influenza pandemic. National Consultative Ethics Committee for Health and Life Sciences. Available at: https://www.ccne-ethique.fr/sites/default/files/publications/avis_106_anglais.pdf.

Amer, A.B., 2019. The ethics of veracity and it is importance in the medical ethics. Open J. Nurs. 9 (2), 194–198.

Armstrong, A., 2007. Nursing ethics: a virtue-based approach. Springer, Basingstoke.

Association for Improvements in the Maternity Services (AIMS), 2012. Top tips for what women want from their midwives. Available at: https://www.aims.org.uk/assets/media/10/aims-top-ten-tips.pdf.

Ballantyne, A., Goold, I., Pearn, A., 2006. Medical genetic services in developing countries: the ethical, legal and social implications of genetic testing and screening. World Health Organization, Switzerland.

Barber, K., 2012. The complexity of decision-making in midwifery: A case study. Br. J. Midwifery 20 (4), 289–294.

Barnfather, T., 2013. Can intuitive knowledge be taught in midwifery practice? Br. J. Midwifery 21 (2), 131–136.

Barrow, J.M., Khandhar, P.B., 2021. Deontology StatPearls [Internet]. StatPearls Publishing, Treasure Island (FL), 2022 Jan–. PMID: 29083671.

Beauchamp, T.L., 2007. The 'four principles' approach to health care ethics. Princ. Health Care Ethics 29, 3–10.

Beauchamp, T.L., Childress, J.F., 2009. Principles of Biomedical Ethics, sixth ed. Oxford University Press, Oxford, England.

Beauchamp, T.L., Childress, J.F., 2013. Principles of Bioethics, seventh ed. Oxford University Press, New York.

Bekker, H.L., 2006. Genetic Screening: Genetic Screening: Facilitating Informed Choices. Encyclopedia of life sciences, pp. 1–5.

Better, S., 2008. Institutional Racism: a Primer on Theory and Strategies for Social Change. Rowman and Littlefield, Lanham.

Braithwaite, J., Travaglia, J.F., 2008. An overview of clinical governance policies, practices and initiatives. Aust. Health Rev. 32 (1), 10–22.

Burgoon, J.K., 1982. Privacy and communication. Ann. Int. Commun. Assoc 6 (1), 206–249.

Camerini, A.L., Schulz, P.J., 2016. Patients' need for information provision and perceived participation in decision making in doctor-patient consultation: Micro-cultural differences between French-and Italian-speaking Switzerland. Patient Educ. Couns. 99 (3), 462–469.

Carlson, G.J., Kordas, K., Murray-Kolb, L.E., 2015. Associations between women's autonomy and child nutritional status: a review of the literature. Matern Child Nutr. 11 (4), 452–482.

Chirkov, V., 2017. Culture and autonomy. In: Church, A.T. (Ed.). The Praeger Handbook of Personality Across Cultures, vol. 2. Praeger, Santa Barbara, CA, pp. 91–101.

Chukwuneke, F.N., Umeora, O.U.J., Maduabuchi, J.U., Egbunike, N., 2014. Global bioethics and culture in a pluralistic world: How does culture influence bioethics in Africa? Ann. Med. Health Sci. Res. 4 (5), 672–675.

Cheyne, H., Dalgleish, L., Tucker, J., Kane, F., Shetty, A., McLeod, S., Niven, C., 2012. Risk assessment and decision making about in-labour transfer from rural maternity care: A social judgment and signal detection analysis. BMC Med. Inform. Decis. Mak. 12 (1), 1–13.

Cholbi, M., 2015. Kant on euthanasia and the duty to die: clearing the air. J. Med. Ethics 41 (8), 607–610.

Christine, P.J., Kaldjian, L.C., 2013. Communicating evidence in shared decision making. AMA J. Ethics 15 (1), 9–17.

Cole, N., 2020. Definition of Cultural Relativism in Sociology. ThoughtCo. Available at: https://www.thoughtco.com/cultural-relativism-definition-3026122 (accessed April 22, 2021).

Cooke, P., 2005. Helping women to make their own decisions. Decision Making in Midwifery Practice, pp. 127–141.

Cullity, G., 2011. Moral judgement The Routledge Encyclopedia of Philosophy. Taylor and Francis., Retrieved 17 Dec. 2021. Available at: https://www.rep.routledge.com/articles/thematic/moral-judgement/v-2.

Curtin, L.L., 1979. The nurse as advocate: a philosophical foundation for nursing. ANS Adv Nurs Sci. 1 (3), 1–10.

Daemers, D.O., van Limbeek, E.B., Wijnen, H.A., Nieuwenhuijze, M.J., de Vries, R.G., 2017. Factors influencing the clinical decision-making of midwives: a qualitative study. BMC Pregnancy Childbirth 17 (1), 345.

Danis, M., Wilson, Y., White, A., 2016. Bioethicists can and should contribute to addressing racism. Am. J. Bioeth. 16 (4), 3–12.

Davies, H.T.O., Mannion, R., Jacobs, R., Powell, A.E., Marshall, M.N., 2007. Exploring the relationship between senior management team culture and hospital performance. Med. Care Res. Rev. 64 (1), 46–65.

Di Mattia, P., 2008. Ethics and culture. In: Kirch, W. (Ed.), Encyclopedia of Public Health. Springer, Dordrecht. Available at: https://doi.org/10.1007/978-1-4020-5614-7_1046.

Dimopoulos, G., 2021. A theory of children's decisional privacy. Legal Studies, pp. 1–24.

Donnelly, J., 1984. Cultural relativism and universal human rights. Hum. Rts. Q. 6, 400.

Draper, E.S., Kurinczuk, J.J., Kenyon, S. (Eds.), 2015. on behalf of MBRRACE-UK, MBRRACE-UK perinatal confidential enquiry: term, singleton, normally formed, antepartum stillbirth. The infant mortality and morbidity studies. Department of health sciences. University of Leicester, Leicester.

Driver, J., 2011. Consequentialism. Routledge, London.

Drysdale. D., 2020. How the 4 principles of healthcare ethics improve patient care. Available at: https://clipboardhealth.com/how-the-4-principles-of-health-care-ethics-improve-patient-care.

Dudzinski, D.M., 2016. Navigating moral distress using the moral distress map. J. Med. Ethics. 42 (5), 321–324.

Ebenstein, A., 2014. Patrilocality and missing women. Available at SSRN 2422090.

Eklöf, N., Hupli, M., Leino-Kilpi, H., 2015. Nurses' perceptions of working with immigrant patients and interpreters in Finland. Public health nursing 32 (2), 143–150.

Elias, A., Paradies, Y., 2021. The costs of institutional racism and its ethical implications for healthcare. J. Bioeth. Inq 18 (1), 45–58.

Elwyn, G., Frosch, D., Thomson, R., Joseph-Williams, N., Lloyd, A., Kinnersley, P., et al., 2012. Shared decision making: A model for clinical practice. J Gen Intern Med. 27 (10), 1361–1367.

Estroff, S.E., Walker, R.L., 2012. Confidentiality: Concealing 'things shameful to be spoken about'. Virtual Mentor 14 (9), 733.

Finn, R.L., Wright, D., Friedewald, M., 2013. Seven types of privacy European Data Protection: Coming of Age. Springer, Dordrecht, pp. 3–32.

Fowler, D., 2008. Student midwives and accountability: Are mentors good role models? Br. J. Midwifery 16 (2), 100–104.

Fowler, M.D., 1989. Social advocacy. Heart Lung 18 (1), 97–99.

Francis, L.P., 2008. Privacy and confidentiality: The importance of context. Monist. 91 (1), 52–67.

Francis, R., 2010. Independent Inquiry into Care Provided by Mid Staffordshire NHS Foundation Trust January 2005-March 2009, vol. 375. The Stationery Office, London.

Frith, L., Sinclair, M., Vehviläinen-Julkunen, K., Beeckman, K., Loytved, C., Luyben, A., 2014. Organisational culture in maternity care: a scoping review. Evidence Based Midwifery 12 (1), 16–22.

Gillon, R., 1994. Medical ethics: four principles plus attention to scope. BMJ. 309 (6948), 184.

Gillon, R., 2003. Ethics needs principles—four can encompass the rest—and respect for autonomy should be 'first among equals'. J. Med. Ethics 29 (5), 307–312.

Glasgow, J., 2009. Racism as disrespect. Ethics 120 (1), 64–93.

Grant, C., 2002. Whistle blowers: Saints of secular culture. J. Bus. Ethics 39 (4), 391–399.

Griffith, R., 2011. Understanding accountability in midwifery practice: Key concepts. Br. J. Midwifery 19 (5), 327–328.

Gronewold, U., Gold, A., Salterio, S.E., 2013. Reporting self-made errors: The impact of organizational error-management climate and error type. J. Bus. Ethics 117 (1), 189–208.

Guerrier, G., Sicard, D., Brey, P.T., 2012. Informed consent: Cultural differences. Nature 483 (7387), 36.

Haddad, L.M., Geiger, R.A., 2021. Nursing ethical considerations StatPearls [Internet]. StatPearls Publishing, Treasure Island (FL), 2022 Jan–. PMID: 30252310.

Hanks, R., 2008. The lived experience of nursing advocacy. Nursing Ethics 15 (4), 468–477.

Hoop, J.G., DiPasquale, T., Hernandez, J.M., Roberts, L.W., 2008. Ethics and culture in mental health care. Ethics Behav. 18 (4), 353–372.

Human Rights Act, 1998. Available at: https://www.legislation.gov.uk/ukpga/1998/42/contents.

IB Global Politics, 2021. Cultural Relativism and Universal Human Rights. Available at: https://sites.google.com/a/isb.be/isbglobalpolitics/unit-human-rights/cultural-relativism-and-universal-human-rights.

ICM., 2018. ICM definitions. Available at: https://www.internationalmidwives.org/our-work/policy-and-practice/icm-definitions.html.

Jayachandran, S., 2015. The roots of gender inequality in developing countries. Economics 7 (1), 63–88.

Jefford, E., 2012. Optimal midwifery decision-making during 2nd stage labour: The integration of clinical reasoning into midwifery practice (Doctoral dissertation, Southern Cross University). NSW, Lismore.

Jefford, E., Jomeen, J., Martin, C.R., 2016. Determining the psychometric properties of the Enhancing Decision-making Assessment in Midwifery (EDAM) measure in a cross cultural context. BMC Pregnancy Childbirth 16 (1), 1–11.

Jenkinson, B., Kruske, S., Stapleton, H., Beckmann, M., Reynolds, M., Kildea, S., 2016. Women's, midwives' and obstetricians' experiences of a structured process to document refusal of recommended maternity care. Women Birth 29 (6), 531–541.

Jones, S.R., 2005. Making ethical decisions Decision making in midwifery practice. Churchill Livingstone, pp. 101–112.

Kao, A., 2002. Seven minutes to midnight. AMA Journal of Ethics. Virtual Mentor. 4 (4). Available at: https://journalofethics.ama-assn.org/article/seven-minutes-midnight/2002-04.

Kirkup, B., 2015. Report of the Morecombe Bay Investigation. Available at: https://assets.publishing.service.gov.uk/government/uploads/system/uploads/attachment_data/file/408480/47487_MBI_Accessible_v0.1.pdf.

Kitchener, K.S., 2000. Foundations of ethical practice research, and teaching in psychology. Lawrence Erlbaum Associates Publishers, Mahwah, NJ.

Kline, A.D., 2006. On complicity theory. Sci. Eng. Ethics 12 (2), 257–264.

Knight, M., Tuffnell, D., Kenyon, S., Shakespeare, J., Gray, R., Kurinczuk, J.J., 2015. Saving lives, improving mothers' care: surveillance of maternal deaths in the UK 2011-13 and lessons learned to inform maternity care from the UK and Ireland. confidential enquiries into maternal deaths and morbidity 2009-13. National Perinatal Epidemiology Unit, University of Oxford.

Kranak, J., 2019. Kantian Deontology. In: Matthews, G. (Ed.), Introduction to Philosophy. Ethics. Available at: https://press.rebus.community/intro-to-phil-ethics/chapter/kantian-deontology/.

Kruske, S., Young, K., Jenkinson, B., Catchlove, A., 2013. Maternity care providers' perceptions of women's autonomy and the law. BMC Pregnancy Childbirth 13 (1), 1–6.

Kubsch, S.M., Sternard, M.J., Hovarter, R., Matzke, V., 2004. A holistic model of advocacy: factors that influence its use. Complement. Ther. Nurs. Midwifery 10 (1), 37–45.

Lachman, V.D., 2008. Whistleblowers: Troublemakers or virtuous nurses. Dermatol. Nurs. 20 (5), 390–393.

Laidsaar-Powell, R., Butow, P., Bu, S., Charles, C., Gafni, A., Fisher, A., Juraskova, I., 2016. Family involvement in cancer treatment decision-making: A qualitative study of patient, family, and clinician attitudes and experiences. Patient Educ. Couns. 99 (7), 1146–1155.

Leino-Kilpi, H., 2000. Patient's Autonomy, Privacy and Informed Consent, vol. 40. IOS press, Amsterdam.

Leino-Kilpi, H., Välimäki, M., Dassen, T., Gasull, M., Lemonidou, C., Scott, A., Arndt, M., 2001. Privacy: a review of the literature. Int J. Nurs. Stud. 38 (6), 663–671.

Lepping, P., Palmstierna, T., Raveesh, B.N., 2016. Paternalism v. autonomy – are we barking up the wrong tree? Br. J. Psychiatry 209 (2), 95–96.

Li, X., 2007. A cultural critique of cultural relativism. Am. J. Econ. Sociol. 66 (1), 151–171.

Lim, G.H.T., Sibanda, Z., Erhabor, J., Bandyopadhyay, S., 2021. Students' perceptions on race in medical education and healthcare. Perspect. Med. Educ. 10 (2), 130–134.

Lindebaum, D., 2012. I Rebel – Therefore we exist: emotional standardization in organizations and the emotionally intelligent individual. J. Manag. Inq. 21 (3), 262–277. https://doi.org/10.1177/1056492611430125.

Lindebaum, D., Geddes, D., Gabriel, Y., 2017. Moral emotions and ethics in organisations: Introduction to the special issue. J. Bus. Ethics 141 (4), 645–656.

Lothian, J.A., 2009. Ethics and maternity care: from principles to practice. J Perinat Educ. 18 (1), 1–3.

Louw, B., 2016. Cultural competence and ethical decision making for health care professionals. Humanities and Social Sciences 4 (2), 41.

Low, L.P.L., Lee, D.T.F., Chan, A.W.Y., 2007. An exploratory study of Chinese older people's perceptions of privacy in residential care homes. J. Adv. Nurs. 57 (6), 605–613.

Lupton, B., Warren, R., 2018. Managing without blame? Insights from the philosophy of blame. J. Bus. Ethics 152 (1), 41–52.

Maina, I.W., Belton, T.D., Ginzberg, S., Singh, A., Johnson, T.J., 2018. A decade of studying implicit racial/ethnic bias in healthcare providers using the implicit association test. Soc. Sci. Med. 199, 219–229.

Mandal, J., Ponnambath, D.K., Parija, S.C., 2016. Utilitarian and deontological ethics in medicine. Trop. Parasitol. 6 (1), 5–7.

Mannion, R., Davies, H., 2018. Understanding organisational culture for healthcare quality improvement. BMJ 363, k4907.

Martin, T., 2015. Law and ethics: a midwifery dilemma. MIDIRS Midwifery Digest 25 (4), 424–429.

Mason, J.K., Laurie, G.T., 2013. Mason and McCall Smith's Law and Medical. Ethics. Oxford University Press, USA.

Mental Capacity Act 2005, c. 9. Available at: http://www.legislation.gov.uk/ukpga/2005/9/contents.

Minkoff, H., 2014. Teaching ethics: when respect for autonomy and cultural sensitivity collide. Am. J. Obstet. Gynecol. 210 (4), 298–301.

Misselbrook, D., 2013. Duty, Kant, and deontology. Br. J. Gen. Pract. 63 (609), 211.

Muaygil, R.A., 2018, March. From paternalistic to patronizing: How cultural competence can be ethically problematic. In: HEC Forum (Vol. 30, No. 1, pp. 13-29). Springer, Netherlands.

Muoni, T., 2012. Decision-making, intuition, and the midwife: understanding heuristics. Br. J. Midwifery 20 (1), 52–56.

Murgic, L., Hébert, P.C., Sovic, S., Pavlekovic, G., 2015. Paternalism and autonomy: Views of patients and providers in a transitional (post-communist) country. BMC Med. Ethics 16 (1), 1–9.

Musalo, K., 2015. When rights and culture collide. Available at: https://www.scu.edu/ethics/ethics-resources/ethical-decision-making/when-rights-and-cultures-collide/.

Naftalin, J., Bewley, S., 2015. Mandatory reporting of FGM. Br. J. Gen. Pract. 65 (638), 450.

Newnham, E., Kirkham, M., 2019. Beyond autonomy: Care ethics for midwifery and the humanization of birth. Nurs. Ethics 26 (7–8), 2147–2157.

NHS., 2003. Confidentiality NHS Code of Practice. Available at: https://assets.publishing.service.gov.uk/government/uploads/system/uploads/attachment_data/file/200146/Confidentiality_-_NHS_Code_of_Practice.pdf.

NHS England., 2020. Female genital mutilation. https://www.england.nhs.uk/north/wp-content/uploads/sites/5/2016/01/fgm-hp-guide.pdf.

NICE., 2017. Shared decision making. Available at: https://www.nice.org.uk/about/what-we-do/our-programmes/nice-guidance/nice-guidelines/shared-decision-making.

NICE., 2021. Overview: antenatal care: guidance. Available at: https://www.nice.org.uk/guidance/NG201.

Nieuwenhuijze, M.J., Low, L.K., Korstjens, I., Lagro-Janssen, T., 2014. The role of maternity care providers in promoting shared decision making regarding birthing positions during the second stage of labor. J. Midwifery Womens Health 59 (3), 277–285.

Nolan, M., 2011. Home birth: the politics of difficult choices. Routledge, London.

Norman, I., 2015. Blind trust in the care-giver: is paternalism essential to the health-seeking behavior of patients in Sub-Saharan Africa? Adv. Appl. Sociol. 5 (2), 94.

Nursing and Midwifery Council (NMC), 2018. The code: professional standards of practice and behaviour for nurses and midwives. NMC, London, Available at. https://www.nmc.org.uk/standards/code/read-the-code-online/.

Ockenden, D., 2020. Emerging Findings and Recommendations from the Independent Review of Maternity Services at The Shrewsbury and Telford Hospital NHS Trust. https://www.donnaockenden.com/downloads/news/2020/12/ockenden-report.pdf.

O'Gorman, C.S., Macken, A.P., Cullen, W., Dunne, C.P., Higgins, M.F., 2013. What is the difference between deontological and consequentialist theories of medical ethics? Ir Med J 106 (2 Suppl), 15–16.

Ogston-Tuck, S., 2014. Ethical issues in palliative and end of life care. In: Nicol, J., Nyatanga, B. (Eds.), Palliative and End of Life Care. Learning, London.

Olsson, A., Adolfsson, A., 2012. Midwife's experiences of using intuition as a motivating element in conveying assurance and care. MIDIRS Midwifery Digest 22 (1), 19–20.

Osamor, P.E., Grady, C., 2016. Women's autonomy in health care decision-making in developing countries: A synthesis of the literature. Int. J. Womens Dermatol. 8, 191.

Park, M.S.A., Chirkov, V., 2020. Culture, Self, and Autonomy. Front. Psychol. 11, 736.

Patrick, K., 2012. Barriers to whistleblowing in the NHS. BMJ, 345.

Provera, B., Montefusco, A., Canato, A., 2010. A'no blame approach to organizational learning. Br. J. Manag. 21 (4), 1057–1074.

Rauwolf, P., Jones, A., 2019. Exploring the utility of internal whistleblowing in healthcare via agent-based models. BMJ Open 9, e021705. https://doi.org/10.1136/bmjopen-2018-021705.

Reichert, E., 2011. Human rights in social work: an essential basis. J. Comp. Soc. Welf. 27 (3), 207–220.

Reichert, E., 2015. Human rights and social work. In: James, D. (Ed.), Wright, International Encyclopedia of the Social & Behavioral Sciences, second ed. Elsevier, pp. 353–359.

Reiger, K., 2008. Domination or mutual recognition? Professional subjectivity in midwifery and obstetrics. Soc. Theory Health 6 (2), 132–147.

Robertson, J.H., Thomson, A.M., 2016. An exploration of the effects of clinical negligence litigation on the practice of midwives in England: A phenomenological study. Midwifery 33, 55–63.

Rosenberg, A.R., Starks, H., Unguru, Y., Feudtner, C., Diekema, D., 2017. Truth Telling in the Setting of Cultural Differences and Incurable Pediatric Illness: A Review. JAMA Pediatr. 171 (11), 1113–1119. https://doi.org/10.1001/jamapediatrics.2017.2568.

Sandman, L., Munthe, C., 2010. Shared decision making, paternalism and patient choice. Health Care Anal. 18 (1), 60–84.

Schilling, J., Kluge, A., 2009. Barriers to organizational learning: an integration of theory and research. Int. J. Manag. Rev. 11 (3), 337–360.

Segal, B.A., Hodges, M., 2012. Care across cultures: Does every patient need to know? Health Prog. 93 (2), 30–35.

Selekman, J., Zavadivker, P., 2021. People of Jewish heritage Textbook for Transcultural Health Care: A Population Approach. Springer, Cham, pp. 557–588.

Senarath, U., Gunawardena, N.S., 2009. Women's autonomy in decision making for health care in South Asia. Asia Pac J Public Health 21 (2), 137–143.

Serenko, N., Fan, L., 2013. Patients' perceptions of privacy and their outcomes in healthcare. Int. J. Behav. Healthc. Res. 4 (2), 101–122.

Showalter, J.S., 2012. The Law of Healthcare Administration. Health Administration Press, Chicago.

Silva, D.S., Gibson, J.L., Sibbald, R., Connolly, E., Singer, P.A., 2008. Clinical ethicists' perspectives on organisational ethics in healthcare organisations. J. Med. Ethics 34 (5), 320–323.

Sonmezer, E., 2021. Professional autonomy for midwives in the contemporary UK maternity system: Part 2. Br. J. Midwifery 29 (1), 19–25.

Sorrell, J.M., 2017. Ethics: Ethical issues with medical errors: shaping a culture of safety in healthcare. Online J. Issues Nurs. 22 (2).

Spaeth, G.L., 2010. Informed choice versus informed consent. Hektoen Int. 2 (2).

Stacey, D., Murray, M.A., Légaré, F., Sandy, D., Menard, P., O'Connor, A., 2008. Decision coaching to support shared decision making: A framework, evidence, and implications for nursing practice, education, and policy. Worldviews Evid. Based Nurs. 5 (1), 25–35.

Sullivan, L.S., 2016. Medical maternalism: beyond paternalism and antipaternalism. J. Med. Ethics 42 (7), 439–444.

Summers, J.W., 1985. Review of nursing practice: the ethical issues, by A. Jameton. Bus. Prof. Ethics J 4 (1), 83–87. Available at: http://www.jstor.org/stable/27799853.

Tai, M.C., Lin, C.S., 2001. Developing a culturally relevant bioethics for Asian people. J. Med. Ethics 27, 51–54.

Tai, M.C.T., Tsai, T.P., 2003. Who makes the decision? Patient's autonomy vs paternalism in a Confucian society. Croat. Med. J. 44 (5), 558–561.

Taj, R., Khan, A., 2018. Importance of bioethics in healthcare. PJNS 13 (1), 4–5.

Taylor, H., 2013. Determining capacity to consent to treatment. Nurs. Times 109 (43), 12–14.

Thompson, A., 2013. Midwives experiences of caring for women who requests are not within clinical policies and guidelines. Br. J. Midwifery 21 (8), 564–570.

Tiran, D., 2012. Bailliere's Midwives' Dictionary E-Book. Elsevier Health Sciences, Edinburgh.

Varkey, B., 2021. Principles of clinical ethics and their application to practice. Med. Princ. Pract. 30 (1), 17–28.

Velasquez, M., Andre, C., Shanks, T., Meyer, S.J., Meyer, M.J., 2014. Justice and Fairness. Available at: https://www.scu.edu/ethics/ethics-resources/ethical-decision-making/justice-and-fairness/.

Watson, C.L., O'Connor, T., 2017. Legislating for advocacy: The case of whistleblowing. Nurs. Ethics 24 (3), 305–312.

Yeung, C.W., 2017. The ethics of collusion and nondisclosure in cancer care: a perspective from professional psychology. Prof. Psychol. Res. Pract. 48 (1), 46.

Zhang, Z., Min, X., 2020. The ethical dilemma of truth-telling in healthcare in China. Journal of bioethical inquiry. 17 (3), 337–344.

Accountability: Being responsible for one's decisions, actions, inactions and omissions.

Acculturation: Cultural modification of an individual, group, or people by adapting to or borrowing traits from another culture; a merging of cultures resulting from prolonged contact. It should be noted that individuals from culturally diverse groups may desire varying degrees of acculturation into the dominant culture.

Advocacy: A means of empowering people by supporting them to assert their views and claim their entitlements and, where necessary, representing and negotiating on their behalf.

Assimilation: To assume the cultural traditions of a given people or group, the cultural absorption of a minority group into the main cultural body.

Asylum seeker: A woman who flees from perceived risk enters a host country and informs the authorities that she wishes to claim asylum.

Autonomy: Most often taken to refer to the ability of an individual to be their own person, to make their own choices based on their own motivations, without manipulation by external forces.

Beneficence: Principle requiring that governments, healthcare providers and researchers do good for, provide benefit to, or make a positive contribution to the welfare of populations, patients and study participants.

Blame culture: An environment where people, or groups/teams of people, are frequently singled out and blamed, criticised and fault is apportioned for mistakes and errors.

Capacity: The ability to understand, deliberate and communicate a choice about a particular healthcare decision at a particular time.

Collectivism: Individualism/Collectivism is one of the Hofstede dimensions in intercultural communication studies. 'Collectivism pertains to societies in which people from birth onwards are integrated into strong, cohesive in-groups, which throughout people's lifetime continue to protect them in exchange for unquestioning loyalty."

Confidentiality: The obligation to keep information secret unless its disclosure has been appropriately authorised by the person concerned or, in extraordinary circumstances, by the appropriate authorities.

Consequentialism: An ethical theory stating that judgement for one's conduct is dependent on the consequences. Therefore, a morally right act has a good outcome.

Culturally appropriate: Exhibiting sensitivity to cultural differences and similarities and demonstrating effectiveness in translating that sensitivity to action through organisational mission statements, communication strategies and services to diverse cultures.

Cultural awareness: Recognition of the nuances of one's own and other cultures.

Cultural beliefs: Beliefs that are learned and shared across groups of people.

Cultural bias: Preference for a particular culture, values, beliefs and norms. Often within an accompanying belief that it is the correct perspective and must guide the situation of decisions.

Cultural competence: The ability of individuals to use academic, experiential and interpersonal skills to increase their understanding and appreciation of cultural differences and similarities within, among and between groups. Cultural competency implies a state of mastery that can be achieved when it comes to understanding culture. Encompasses individuals' desire, willingness and ability to improve systems by drawing on diverse values, traditions and customs and working closely with knowledgeable persons from the community to develop interventions and services that affirm and reflect the value of different cultures.

Cultural desire: The motivation of the healthcare professional to 'want to' engage in the process of becoming culturally aware, culturally knowledgeable, culturally skilful and seeking cultural encounters; not the 'have to'.

Cultural diversity: Differences in race, ethnicity, nationality, religion, gender, sexual identity, socioeconomic status, physical ability, language, beliefs, values, behaviour patterns or customs among various groups within a community, organisation or nation.

Cultural encounters: A process that encourages the healthcare professional to engage directly in face-to-face cultural interactions and other types of encounters with clients from culturally diverse backgrounds to modify existing beliefs about a cultural group and prevent possible stereotyping.

Cultural humility: A lifelong process of self-reflection and self-critique. Cultural humility does not require mastery of lists of 'different' or peculiar beliefs and behaviours supposedly pertaining to different cultures; instead, it encourages developing a respectful attitude towards diverse points of view.

Cultural norms: The agreed-upon expectations and rules by which a culture guides the behaviour of its members in any given situation

Cultural relativism: The ability to understand a **culture** on its own terms and not to make judgements using the standards of one's own **culture**.

Cultural rituals: A patterned, repetitive and symbolic enactment of a cultural belief or value.

Cultural safety: A concept that focuses on culturally appropriate healthcare services, as well as improving healthcare access, inequalities in health, unequal power relations and the social, political and historical context of care

Cultural sensitivity: Understanding the needs and emotions of your own culture and the culture of others.

Cultural skill: The ability to collect culturally relevant data regarding the patient's presenting problem, as well as accurately performing culturally based physical, spiritual, psychological and medication assessments in a culturally sensitive manner.

Cultural values: The individual's desirable or preferred way of acting or knowing something that is sustained over time and that governs actions.

Culture: An integrated pattern of human behaviour that includes thoughts, communications, languages, practices, beliefs, values, customs, courtesies, rituals, manners of interacting, roles, relationships and expected behaviours of a racial, ethnic, religious or social group; the ability to transmit the above to succeeding generations; culture is constantly changing.

Culture shock: A state of distress and tension with possible physical symptoms after a person relocates to an unfamiliar cultural environment.

Decisional conflict: Personal uncertainty about which course of action to take when choice among competing options involves risk, regret or challenge to personal life values

Deontology: A theory that states that actions are good or bad according to a set of rules.

Discrimination: A prejudiced or prejudicial outlook, action or treatment (e.g., racial discrimination).

Duty of care: An obligation to perform to a certain standard of conduct to protect another against an unreasonable risk of harm.

Enculturation: The sociological process of raising a child to be a member of a particular culture or cultural group.

Ethics: Branch of knowledge concerned with questions about right versus wrong conduct and what constitutes a good or bad life, as well as the justificatory basis for such questions.

Ethnic: Of or relating to large groups of people classed according to common racial, national, tribal, religious, linguistic, or cultural origin or background.

Ethnic group: Group characterised by cultural similarities (shared among members of that group) and differences (between that group and others). Members of an ethnic group share beliefs, values, habits, customs, norms, a common language, religion, history, geography, kinship and/or race.

Ethnocentrism: The tendency that people have to evaluate others from their own cultural reference.

Evidence-based practice: An authorised/agreed change in the role of an individual registered nurse or registered midwife to include areas of practice that have not previously been within their scope of practice but are within the overall scope of practice of the nursing and midwifery professions.

Fidelity: Means to care for women with consideration, loyalty, caring and honesty.

Harm: Any deliberate or accidental physical, emotional, psychological, social or reputational injury or damage to a person's health or to any other party or parties to whom a duty of care is owed.

Health literacy: The degree to which individuals can obtain, process and understand basic health information and services needed to make appropriate health decisions.

Immigrants: People who voluntarily move to a country of which they are not natives to take up permanent residence.

Individualism: Individualism/Collectivism is one of the Hofstede dimensions in intercultural communication studies. He defines this dimension as: 'Individualism pertains to societies in which the ties between individuals are loose: everyone is expected to look after himself or her-self and his or her immediate family'.

Informed choice: A process of decision-making involving a partnership between a woman and her midwife, based on the underlying assumption that women have a right to receive accurate, non-biased information and then make an informed acceptance or refusal, knowing that the midwife will respect her choice.

Informed consent: Agreement to a certain course of action, such as treatment or participation in research, based on complete and relevant information by a competent individual without coercion.

Intuitive decision-making: The process by which information acquired through associated learning and stored in long-term memory is accessed unconsciously to form the basis of a judgement or decision.

Justice: A highly contested concept that can roughly be thought of as giving people what they deserve.

Marginalisation: The practice of excluding a social group from the mainstream of the society, placing that group legally or socially on the 'margins' of the society.

Maternal morbidity: Any physical or mental illness or disability directly related to pregnancy and/or childbirth. These are not necessarily life-threatening but can have a significant impact on the quality of life.

Maternal mortality: The death of a woman while pregnant or within 42 days of termination of pregnancy, irrespective of the duration and site of the pregnancy, from any cause related to or aggravated by the pregnancy or its management but not from accidental or incidental causes.

Microaggressions: A word used to describe everyday subtle remarks or actions that are insulting to marginalised groups.

Morals: Values that we attribute to a system of beliefs that help the individual define right versus wrong, good versus bad. These typically get their authority from something outside the individual—a higher being or higher authority (e.g., government, society).

Moral absolutism: The belief there are universal ethical standards that apply to every situation.

Moral dilemma: A situation in which the decision-maker must consider two or more moral values or duties but can only honour one of them.

Moral distress: The emotional state that arises from a situation when a person feels that the ethically correct action to take is different from what they are tasked with doing.

Moral uncertainty: The inability to determine the 'right' course of moral action to pursue.

Moral universalism: Is the concept that moral principles are universal and apply to everyone, regardless of culture, ethnicity, race, religion or gender.

Nonmaleficence: A principle requiring that healthcare providers and researchers do not inflict undue harm, either intentionally or through negligence.

Paralanguage: The non-verbal elements of communication used to modify meaning and convey emotion. Paralanguage may be expressed consciously or unconsciously, and it includes the pitch, volume and, in some cases, intonation of speech.

Prejudice: Uninformed judgements about others that are often unconscious, harsh or discriminatory and that involve rejection.

Principlism: An applied ethics approach to the examination of moral dilemmas that is based upon the application of certain ethical principles.

Privacy: Privacy seeks to protect a person from scrutiny by others. Respect for privacy implies that a person should not be expected to share personal information unless they choose. Any violation of privacy requires ethical justification.

Race: There is an array of different beliefs about the definition of race and what race means within social, political and biological contexts. The following definitions are representative of these perspectives:

A tribe, people or nation belonging to the same stock; a division of humankind possessing traits that are transmissible by descent and sufficient to characterise it as a distinctive human type.

Racism: Theories, attitudes and practices that display dislike or antagonism towards people seen as belonging to particular ethnic groups. Social or political significance is attached to culturally constructed ideas of difference.

Refugees: People who migrate because of political oppression or war usually with legal permission to stay in a different country.

Rite of passage: Any life cycle rite that marks a person's or group's transition from one social state to another.

Ritual: A repeatable, often customary action with deep meaning and significance by which persons express and reinforce relationships among themselves or with God; considered a constitutive element of culture.

Safety culture: A combination of the attitudes, values and perceptions that influence *how* something is done in the workplace, rather than *how it should be* done.

Stereotypes: Unsubstantiated beliefs about the personal attributes of the members of a group based on inaccurate generalisations that are used to describe all members of the group and that thus ignore individual differences.

Stigma: A term describing the condition of possessing an identity that has been branded 'spoiled' or discredited identity by others. Examples of negative social stigmas are physical or mental handicaps and disorders and homosexuality or affiliation with a specific nationality, religion or ethnicity.

Systemic racism: Also known as institutional racism, is a form of racism embedded through laws within society or an organisation.

Tradition: The handing down of information, beliefs and customs by word of mouth or by example from one generation to another without written instruction.

Traditional Medicine: Medicine and healthcare practices which originated in a particular culture and have been practised by an ethnic or cultural group for centuries in the country of origin or of emigration.

Unconscious bias: Unconscious bias is prejudice favouring or against a person or group of people against another negatively or unfairly.

Utilitarianism: A version of consequentialism states that an ethical decision is right or wrong depending on the consequences.

Values: The core beliefs we hold regarding what is right and fair in terms of our actions and our interactions with others. Another way to characterise values is that they are what an individual believes to be of worth and importance to their life (valuable). (From 'What is the Difference Between Ethics, Morals and Values?', Frank Navran.)

Veracity: The process of being honest and telling the truth and is related to the principle of autonomy. It is the basis of the trust relationship established between a patient and a healthcare provider.

Whistleblowing: The act of disclosing information about wrongdoing in the workplace.

C